"HELP LORD—
THE DEVIL WANTS ME FAT!"

ABOUT THE AUTHOR

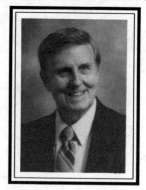

DR. C. S. LOVETT

Dr. Lovett is the president of **Personal Christianity,** a fundamental, evangelical interdenominational ministry. For the past 44 years he has had but one objective—**preparing Christians for the second coming of Christ!** This book is one of over 44 of his works designed to help believers **prepare for His appearing.**

Dr. Lovett's decision to serve the Lord resulted in the loss of a sizable personal fortune. He is well equipped for the job the Lord has given him. A graduate of American Baptist Seminary of the West, he holds the **M.A.** and **M.Div.** degrees conferred *Magna Cum Laude.* He has also completed graduate work in psychology at Los Angeles State College and holds a **Ph.D.** in counseling from the Louisiana Christian University.

A retired Air Force Chaplain (Lt. Colonel), he has been married to Marjorie for 53 years and has two grown daughters dedicated to the Lord.

"HELP LORD—
THE DEVIL WANTS ME FAT!"

by C. S. LOVETT
M.A., M.Div., Ph.D.

author of
**DEALING WITH THE DEVIL
JESUS WANTS YOU WELL
SOUL-WINNING MADE EASY
LATEST WORD ON THE LAST DAYS**

president of Personal Christianity

ILLUSTRATED BY LINDA LOVETT

published by
PERSONAL CHRISTIANITY
Baldwin Park, California 91706

ISBN 0-938148-33-8
1995 EDITION

Contents

"HELP LORD—THE DEVIL WANTS ME FAT!"

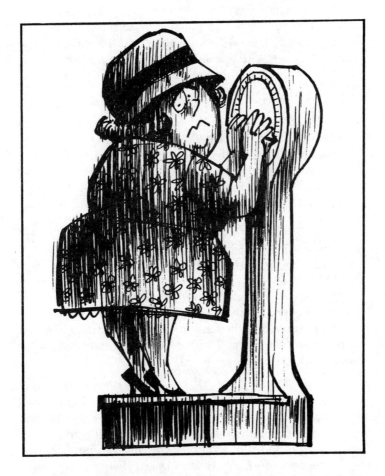

Does that lady make you chuckle? Praise the Lord we can find something humorous in a serious problem. For those overweight, there's nothing funny about being fat. Several years ago I published an article in our monthly newsletter, *CAN THE DEVIL MAKE YOU FAT?* It had to do with Satan's power to make Christians overeat. The response was overwhelming. It pointed up the need for a book that would give God's people **A PLAN for breaking the devil's hold on them through food.**

Most of the letters were outright cries for help. Here beside my typewriter is a stack of selected letters. I'll share two or three with you, then you'll appreciate the motivation behind this book. I won't use their names. That might prove embarrassing. First we hear from Mrs. C. P. of Pennsylvania:

> *"Dear Dr. Lovett, I'm writing in response to your article, 'Can the Devil make you fat?' I'm suffering very much from being overweight. I'm 5 feet 2 inches and weigh 225 pounds. I'm disgusted and depressed. All I want to do is eat constantly. I've sought the Lord's help again and again, but it seems there is no help for me. I'm convinced the devil is doing this. It keeps me from going to church and from being the kind of wife and mother I long to be. I pray God will somehow use you to help me."*

Can you feel her frustration? Wouldn't you want to help someone like that if you could? Now if you're only slightly overweight, her case might seem extreme. Maybe this letter from Mrs. T. S. in California expresses your sentiment better:

> *"I'm 20 years old Dr. Lovett, and I love the Lord very much. But I have a problem with food. Honestly it's a 'thorn' in my side. I'm not really fat, but I'm a compulsive eater. My whole attitude toward food is bad. I'm afraid it sometimes comes between me and the Lord. When I'm not dieting, I'm a glutton. I get control for a time, then I lose it. I'm fighting a losing battle. I need help. I want those*

chains broken. I know the Lord is willing and able to help me, but I need good counsel to get there."

One more letter will give you an idea of the mail that bombarded me, practically forcing me to write this book. It comes from Mrs. D. W. C. in Connecticut:

"Dear Dr. Lovett, I'm desperate for help. I'm quite a bit overweight. I feel terrible about it and look worse. The problem is I can't stick to a diet. Somehow I have fooled myself into believing the excess weight would sort of go away by itself. But now, after 7 years, I'm realizing to my horror that it is getting worse. The effect on my life is devastating. I know it is depleting my Christian witness and energy for the Lord."

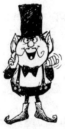 If you were to go through this stack of letters at one sitting, you'd get the feeling that Satan had unleashed **an army of glutton demons** on American Christians. Food is so abundant in our country and comes in such variety, that it can easily be turned into an obsession. When it comes to finding ways to choke off God's power in the lives of His children, the devil doesn't miss a trick. What could be more clever than making an idol out of eating? **It's so respectable, yet it can be just as enslaving as drugs or alcohol.** Passion for food is every bit as consuming as the lust for sex or money or fame.

One reader sent me this note as an urgent message:

"Brother Lovett, there appears to be a satanic plot at work in the land to make Christians obese. You'd do the body of Christ a great service if you'd tell us how to cope with this attack on God's people."

I feel that way myself. As far as I'm concerned, a

satanic food conspiracy is in existence. As a result, a multitude of believers across this country is overloaded with fat. Not only does it make them look ugly, but it drains their energy, and loads up their hearts making them more susceptible to disease—including cancer. Many of them are discouraged. Try as they might, they cannot let food alone. It is a relentless master from which they long to be free. Many of them say they've tried everything to escape the "crippling chains of food addiction," but nothing seems to work. What a setup for Satan. How he delights to whisper in the consciences of his victims . . .

"If the Lord can't give you victory in something as simple as food, how can you expect victory in other areas of your life?"

That hurts. How many, do you suppose, suspect a connection between their overeating and the devil? Very few, you can be sure of that.

SO I HAD TO DO THIS BOOK

If you have read any of my books, you know I specialize in practical helps for the Christian life. The plans you see in those books are largely based on actual experience. Whether it is witnessing or dealing with the devil or healing the body, generally I wait until the Holy Spirit has taken me through the experience personally. Then my friends test what I have written. Finally when we're all satisfied we're giving the Lord the best we have, we put it into print.

That's the way our PC tools are developed.

The book you are reading had its beginnings in my own need. When I began my first experiments, I weighed 205 pounds. That's far too much weight for me to carry. I'm just a shade over 5 feet 10 inches tall. I could feel the squeeze when I bent over to tie my shoes. That tells a man he's in bad shape. But there were other clues as well.

I didn't have the PEP and BOUNCE that go with a trim body. Much of my vitality for Christ was drained off by the extra weight. That in turn sapped much of my joy. So it was time I did something about it. I tried various diet plans. Some were great for getting the weight off. Then I'd forsake the diet and back would come the weight. For several years my weight went up and down like a yo-yo as I tried first one plan then another. Finally, the Lord gave me the program set forth in this book.

I set a goal for myself—170 pounds. That meant I had to lose 35 pounds. Well, those pounds came off easily and quickly. But here's the exciting part—I haven't put them back on. It's easy to keep the weight off by this method. Since I received it from the Lord, I feel it could well be the ULTIMATE WAY to control a person's weight. I'm thrilled with the plan. I thank the Lord for it. I know you're going to like it. So get set for a terrific blessing, because that's what's coming!

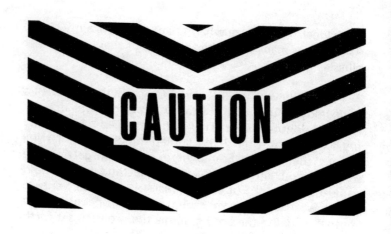

READ THIS SECTION BEFORE
STARTING CHAPTER ONE

"HELP LORD—the devil wants me fat!"

What did you think when you first read the title of this book? Did you identify with the first two words . . . "HELP LORD?" If you're overweight, you probably know by experience how futile are the fad diets and crash programs. You may have tried them all. Help from the Lord may seem like the only answer. It's possible you said to yourself . . . "Maybe there's hope for me at last!"

But how do you feel about the other five words . . . "the devil wants me fat?" Do they bring up your eyebrows? Thinking they might, I have inserted this caution. As you start into the book, you could run into ideas that may not be familiar to you. Or, they might even be repulsive. But don't let that keep you from going all the way and receiving the great blessing and relief this book has for you. It really will bring you help from the Lord.

The first three chapters speak of the devil. I make no apology for that. To me he's as real as the Lord. I'm convinced he plays a strategic part in making us fat and keeping us that way. I realize many shy away from referring to Satan in connection with anything, largely out of superstition, I feel. It's time we came right out and put the blame where it belongs. At the same time I recognize it is possible that referring to the devil as an active personality may be new to you. Or my mention of his having anything to do with our eating habits could turn you off. But don't let that happen.

Don't allow preconceived notions about the devil to keep you from getting the help you need. That's why I hasten to let you know what this book can do for you. **It is a 3-STEP plan for getting your weight off and keeping it off.** It is rooted in basic laws and so powerful I'm sure you won't want to miss it. I know some of my ideas might sound new and strange to you, and for that reason the first three chapters will unfold the part that Satan plays in making us fat. If you have any kind of a weight problem or simply an obsessive desire for food, don't let a disturbing point or two rob you of the blessing God has for you. Bear with me . . . you won't be sorry.

Here's what you can expect from this book.

There are **THREE PHASES** to the approach. What I have to say about Satan has to do with only **ONE** of these phases:

1. First you'll learn **HOW the devil is able to influence our eating.** Also how to recognize his suggestions for getting us to eat more than we should. And beyond that, how to deal with him. You'll get a new picture of Satan's power.

2. **Then you'll learn how to deal with your appetite.** The plan offers a startling way to gain control over your body and put to silence those compulsions which urge you to eat . . . and eat . . . and eat.

3. Finally, and this is the most powerful feature of the plan, you'll learn how to **DE-PROGRAM** yourself from bad eating habits. Then, working with the Lord, you'll harness the POWER of your body's own com-

puter system to make you eat the kinds of foods you should and in the right amounts. You're going to laugh when you see yourself turned off to the very foods you used to love.

Believe me, those three steps offer the most powerful help God has for his people today. So don't choke on the first chapters if the ideas are new to you. Instead, look on them as a challenge. As you read, let the Holy Spirit be the Referee should something sound startling or different. If you can do that, the book will be FUN for you. A new adventure.

Also, you should be watching for interruptions and distractions. The devil will do all he can to hinder your concentration. The reason I tell you about this **in advance,** is because I know it will strengthen your faith when you see things HAPPEN BEFORE YOUR EYES. Satan doesn't want you to come into this kind of knowledge. He knows you'll end up trim and attractive—a real credit to Christ. So watch out for him. When those negative feelings start creeping up on you, recognize their source.

Now get set for a fabulous experience. When it's over, you're going to look different, feel different and be different. It is going to be exciting for you to watch the changes take place in your body as the techniques of this book become yours to use. So let's get into that first chapter and see how it sets on your spirit. You should be ready for it—now.

PHASE ONE

How to
deal with the devil

Please read the CAUTION on page 12 before starting chapter one. If you don't, you might not be prepared for what lies ahead.

The Satanic Food Conspiracy!

"For the spirit that God gave us is no craven spirit, but one to inspire strength, love, and self-discipline." (2 Tim. 1:7 NEB)

"I don't see how a really fat person can be a true Christian!"

Normally I ignore such remarks. We all know that being fat or skinny has nothing to do with being saved. But the brother making the statement was so sincere, I thought I'd better hear him out.

"Oh," I replied, "How come?"

"Well in Philippians 3:19, the apostle Paul speaks of those whose god is their belly. When a person is over-

weight it seems to me that food is his real master, not the Lord Jesus. Those extra pounds are proof he puts his stomach ahead of the Lord."

I'M SURE I REACTED NEGATIVELY

I was overweight at the time. A little sensitive too, I might add. So my first inclination was to argue. Then I remembered something Charles Finney said in his living Bible lectures . . . **"Whenever you see a fat Christian, you're looking at a man who is not walking with the Lord."** That caused me to do some heart-searching. "Was I putting food ahead of the Lord? Did I honor the demands of my tummy before those of Christ?"

Then I looked down at the rolls around my waistline. One thing was obvious—I was eating more food than I needed. Those excess pounds proved it. Ah, but connecting that excess with the Lordship of Christ was new to me. I hadn't met that idea before. "Is it possible the devil was using food to WEAKEN the Lord's rule over my life?" Ugh, I didn't like that idea. Probably because the answer I was getting back was a "yes."

From what I knew of the devil, food was something he would definitely use. He's skillful in turning good things to evil purposes. It's his nature to do so. Take for example, what he does with money. Money is also a necessity. All he has to do is stir up the desire for a LITTLE MORE of it, and thousands of Christians will spend time and talent chasing dollars. Before they know it, making money is more important than serving the Lord. Since a person cannot serve BOTH money and the Lord, it is Jesus who loses out when it's a choice between overtime pay or being in the house of the Lord.

Or we could consider sex.

Here is a beautiful thing God has given us, a drive of the organism to remind us how incomplete we are in ourselves. Just as we need a mate to make us complete in the flesh, so do we need the Lord Jesus to be complete in the spirit (Col. 2:10). But my, how Satan has perverted this glorious gift in our day. We're close to matching the evil of Sodom and Gomorrah. If Satan has the ability to take God-given drives and turn them to evil, why would he ignore something as vital as eating? He doesn't, of course. The need to eat is too powerful a force in our lives for him to overlook. Therefore the desire for food has to be in his bag of tricks.

WE'RE GEARED TO EATING

That's the way God made us. Even though it is possible to go for days without eating, no one can survive indefinitely without food. However, it seems few realize HOW LITTLE of it the body really needs. The body can get along on far less than the average American consumes.

When we're eating, do we think in terms of what our bodies need? No, we think of how good it tastes or how satisfying it is to stuff ourselves. That's got to be the work of Satan. He gets us to shift our focus from eating what we **NEED**, to eating what we **WANT**. He knows that if he can get us to eat ONE BITE MORE than we need, his influence has been effective.

Beyond that, there seems to be a **FOOD CONSPIRACY** in our land. Fast food stands are springing up like gas stations. Household magazines are filled with color photos of delicious pastries and desserts. Everywhere you look it's food—**food**—**FOOD**. The great American pastime is one of eating—**eating**—**EATING**. We're a nation of gluttons!

"Our enemies don't have to attack us. All they need to do is give us all the ice cream we want, and we'll wipe ourselves out"
— Dr. David Pritkin.

I'd say there was a food conspiracy—and it's working!

CHRISTIANS IMMUNE?

Not long after he is saved, the new Christian learns his body is no longer his own. It belongs to the Lord Jesus, having become the **"temple of the Holy Spirit"** (I Cor. 6:19). The apostle Paul says precisely, "The body . . . is for the Lord" (I Cor. 6:13). That being so, it is in his BODY that the Christian should display the Spirit's power. As he submits to the Holy Spirit, he will be led into temperate and moderate use of that body.

Most Christians seem to think it still belongs to them; that they can do with it as they please. As a result they pollute it and defile it. We're familiar with the usual things that defile the body: drugs, alcohol, tobacco and sex sins. James says the uncontrolled tongue also defiles the body. **But most subtle is the way the devil gets us to defile our bodies with food.** Many who profess to put Christ first in their lives, deny His lordship with a knife and fork. If they persist, they soon find they have ANOTHER GOD demanding their time, money and attention.

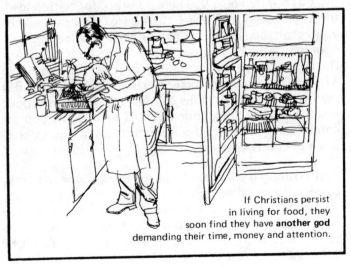

If Christians persist in living for food, they soon find they have **another god** demanding their time, money and attention.

Thus we have Christians who wouldn't think of lying or stealing or committing adultery, unashamedly going around with bulging bellies. By this they are announcing to the world, **"I've got another god in my life!"** This is in direct violation of the First Commandment which says, **"Thou shalt have no other gods before Me!"** The fat Christian has definitely taken up with an idol—FOOD! If it is impossible to serve God and mammon, **it is equally impossible to serve GOD AND FOOD!** There can only be one master and the devil knows it.

It's easy for the devil to make Christians fat. All he has to do is get them to eat a LITTLE MORE than they need. Here's what's so tricky about it. He's not leading us in an **unholy direction.** Food is a necessity. We have to eat. It is something GOD has ordained. The devil merely wants us to eat MORE of something that is good, more than we should. **When we do, we're living to eat, rather than eating to live.** When that becomes our way of life—HE'S GOT US!

SO SIMPLE FOR SATAN

You're watching TV. There's a break for station identification. Do you just sit there? No. You ease out of your chair and head for the kitchen. The refrigerator door swings open. You peer inside. Are you hungry? No. Does your body need food right now? No. Do you know why you're standing there, staring like that? No. But here you are anyway. How come? The devil has dropped the EAT IDEA into your mind. By this time, you are conditioned to respond automatically. You don't challenge the idea—you obey it.

If nothing is available from the refrigerator, you may open a cupboard or two. Some more staring. If you spy something that can be eaten conveniently, you reach for it. If not, you close the door . . . "I don't need it anyway." But that's a victory of the moment. You'll be back shortly. You win sometimes and you lose sometimes, but the final score is totaled up on the bathroom scale. If you've **gained** weight, you are clearly **losing** the war.

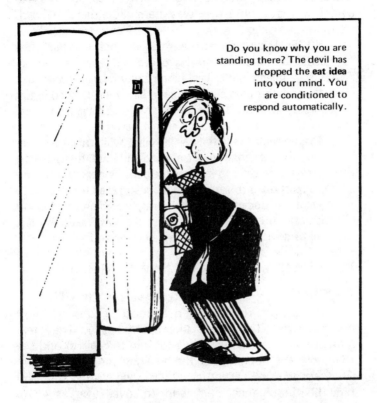

Do you know why you are standing there? The devil has dropped the **eat idea** into your mind. You are conditioned to respond automatically.

The point? **The devil encounters practically no resistance in getting you to eat.**

SATAN AND THE BLUBBER BUSINESS

The devil doesn't care about fat. He's concerned with what happens to Christians **when** they're fat. He knows what it does to people. In spite of the common notion that fat people are more jolly, **the real truth is they are often more lonely.** They make good pals, but not sweethearts. As a result, fat people do a lot of pretending.

Often their romantic life is one big fantasy. And when you consider that Satan is at home in the imagination, it's easy to see how he might turn those fantasies to evil. But that's only one way he afflicts us with food.

> **NOTE.** There are cases where an overweight condition is NOT due to eating of excess food. Some people have glandular problems and can get fat on a survival diet. Fewer than 1% have this problem. **We do not have them in mind in this discussion.** Then there are those who can apparently eat anything and in any amount and never put on a pound. **These people we DO have in mind.** While they may not have the outward evidence of overindulgence, they have the appetite and cater to it. Since the body belongs to the Lord, we must learn to eat and drink as unto the Lord. We are to guard our bodies with a holy fear, lest Satan use them to impose HIS WILL on our lives. We must realize what a subtle door our stomachs provide for the devil.

OTHER REASONS SATAN WANTS US FAT

❶ DESPAIR. How many overweight Christians cry out to the Lord for victory over food? Thousands, you can be sure. They don't like being heavy. They feel guilty about it every time they look in the mirror and see that ugly fat hanging on them. They long to be trim. They spend hard earned money buying clothes that will hide their indulgence. They want to cover it up, as Adam and Eve did to hide their nakedness. In the meantime they pray and pray . . . and nothing comes of it. But WILL the Lord take away their appetite for food as they ask? No. They'd die. The problem is NOT eating, but **over**eating—even if it is but a tiny excess.

Until a Christian dedicates his stomach to the Lord, he can pray all he wants and nothing will happen. The body is the Lord's. And the relationship between the body and the spirit is so close, that the **power of the Holy Spirit in one's life DEPENDS ON THE YIELDING OF THE BODY TO CHRIST.** Frequently the greatest barrier to surrender of the body is the STOMACH. Until it is surrendered, the person can pray until he is blue in the face and there'll be no answer. He prays in disappointment. When his disappointment becomes despair, the devil has acquired a destructive emotion to use against him.

❷ **FOOTHOLD.** What Satan really seeks is a foothold on our WILLS. At first he is satisfied with a tiny bit of control. If he can just get his foot in the door, he knows he can expand his influence. And when we take ONE BITE of food more than we need, it provides him with a chink in our armor, an opening in our defense. When he can get us to eat more than we need—at his suggestion— he has gained the foothold he wants. That is why a few extra pounds is such a serious matter. They become an unanswerable proof of his dominion. Obviously he expects to expand his influence from food to other areas of our lives such as worry and temper and sex. But he is happy to start with that ONE BITE EXTRA.

❸ **ENSLAVEMENT.** This is what the devil is finally after. He doesn't want us in control of our flesh. He wants us SLAVES of our flesh. Why? The flesh is his territory. The fall of Adam made the devil complete master over the realm of the flesh. Our souls have been redeemed, but our bodies are awaiting redemption at the Lord's return (Rom. 8:22,23). Therefore, when we are enslaved to some drive or weakness of the flesh, we become, in effect, **slaves of Satan.** How it thrills him to have a child of God fall into his hands as a slave. He knows it hurts the Lord to see us in bondage. The devil just loves to make fools of the sons of God.

> **NOTE.** Should I make a special point of sluggishness? I'm sure you already know the person who is overweight through self-indulgence, finally ends up with a sluggish SPIRIT. His zip and vitality are drained off by the excess weight. It's easier for him to sink into a sofa and watch TV than to serve the Lord. As things go from bad to worse he

starts putting things off . . . "I can do it tomorrow." He falls into a pattern of procrastination. With his pep and vigor gone, he becomes susceptible to disease—including cancer. It may never enter his head that the devil has used FOOD to do this to him. Think how many have become unfit for service as the devil used their appetites to disqualify them. The fat, sluggish Christian displays in his body the identifying marks of his real master—THE DEVIL!

WHAT GOD THINKS OF IT

I've employed such gentle words as "overeating" and "excess food" in picturing Satan's dominion. I've also said that all he needs to do to make us fat is to get us to eat just a **LITTLE MORE** than we need. One bite more than we need will do it. But the Bible isn't quite that delicate about it. It labels the practice of overeating as **SIN** and gives it the name . . . **GLUTTONY!** This is one sin you don't hear much about. It's as if we'd all gotten together and agreed not to talk about it. But it's time the lid came off. As far as I can determine, we are in those days of "eating and drinking" of which the Lord spoke (Matt. 24:37-39). It is one of the signs of the last days.

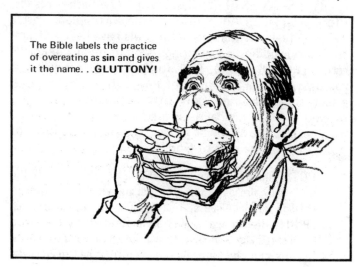

The Bible labels the practice of overeating as **sin** and gives it the name. . .**GLUTTONY!**

I'm looking at a prayer request from a dear brother who was aware of his bondage and calls it what it really is—SIN. He writes:

"Please pray for me. I need release from the sin of overeating. No, let's call it for what it is—GLUTTONY! My heart's desire is that God would use me as a soul-winner and let me serve Him in building soul-winning churches. I want to go all out for Christ, but this sin HAS ME BOUND."

See how this brother recognized the seriousness of the situation? He knew it was beyond his power to free himself. Many do not. For some reason, Christians consider food as utterly harmless, and that being bound by something as innocent as food is somehow acceptable to God. The truth is, **God hates it.** Why? He has already given His children the POWER TO CONTROL THEMSELVES.

 "For the Spirit that God gives us is no craven spirit, but one to inspire strength, love and self-discipline" (2 Tim. 1:7 NEB).

• We believers make a big to do about walking in the Spirit and being LED by the Spirit. When someone has a problem with cigarettes or alcohol or sex, we say . . . **"Tsk, tsk, how awful! He's fallen into Satan's hands."** But we're not really honest in the matter until we get serious about the one area that screams for control— FOOD. For some reason we have come to look on an appetite for sex or liquor as being more offensive to God than an appetite for food. But is that really so? When you come right down to it, it is not the THING that binds us that is offensive to God, but that we are in bondage when we shouldn't be.

 Some years ago a well known evangelist on the West Coast was shot and killed in a motel room by an enraged husband. The preacher was caught in bed with the man's wife. When the story broke in the newscasts, Christians around me gasped in judgment. I recall various ones saying, "What an awful way to meet the Lord!" But let me ask this: "Is it any worse for the Lord to find you in bed with someone else's wife or husband, or to have Him find you 20-50 pounds overweight? Is one any better off than the other when it comes to self-indulgence?

Think about it. What evidence do we have that God views the sex appetite as more criminal than an appetite for food? Earlier in the chapter I named six ways a man can defile his body. Sex sin was only one of them. Is the passion for sex or drink somehow more evil than the passion for food? No. The Bible puts gluttony in the same class as drunkenness and adultery (Deut. 21:20; Rom. 13:13; Gal. 5:19-21; I Pet. 4:3).

IT'S THE BONDAGE GOD HATES

We are the **"temple of the living God"** (2 Cor. 6:16). The body is to be kept holy and used for the Lord. God's Word condemns any appetite that brings us into bondage to Satan. It was by eating that sin and the fall of man came about. It was through eating that Satan sought to tempt the Lord. When we refuse to give Jesus lordship over our stomachs, we give the devil a way to bind us. It matters little to the Lord WHICH appetite the devil uses—it's the bondage He hates.

When a man is bound in chains, does it matter to him whether those chains are made of gold, or iron, steel or aluminum? He's still bound. Slavery is slavery, whether it is to drink, sex or food. Without our being aware of it, the devil moves silently into life after life, so that almost every Christian has been invaded at the food frontier.

Wouldn't you agree that it's time we took note of what he is doing and put an end to it? Of course you do.

28

You wouldn't be reading this book if you didn't. Well here's good news. The Lord has given us powerful weapons for dealing with the devil—and the authority to use them. Beyond that, His Word sets forth a fantastic way to regain control of our bodies. When that happens, the Christian experiences the power of the Holy Spirit in a remarkable way.

SUMMARY

Everywhere you look you see fat Christians. In some places they make jokes about it. But to the believer with the bulging belly it is no joke. He's over his head, bound by something he can't handle. He looks at those rolls around his waistline, ashamed to feel so helpless in the face of food. Inwardly, it's embarrassing for him to have the proof of his weakness and lack of self-control hanging out there for anyone to see. He knows what they're thinking.

But does it ever occur to him that an outside force may be responsible? Not unless he has been taught about the devil. He'll blush and bear it, not realizing that he is a victim of Satan. Isn't that sad? How many must be in that same plight? **The plain fact is the devil IS responsible.** He works behind the scenes getting Christians to eat more than they need, yet who suspects he has anything to do with it? If he can get them to take **ONE BITE** more than they need, he's got his foot in the door. Before long he has them ENSLAVED, living to eat rather than eating to live.

Gluttony is a sin we don't talk about because we don't realize the devil's part in it. If we did, we wouldn't hesitate to put it where it belongs . . . right along with drunkenness and adultery. It's hard for the devil to tempt the spiritual Christian with drink and dope and sex, so he has to resort to more subtle things . . . **like food.** The man who can't be tempted into adultery, might easily be led into overeating . . . because food is so innocent looking. But as far as God is concerned, one form of bondage is as bad as another. And to see one of His servants with a bulging belly, is just as bad as seeing him in bed with another's wife.

29

It's time we all started learning how the devil works to destroy us with food. Before we can deal with him, to get him off our backs, we need to learn just how it is he makes us eat. That's next.

CHAPTER TWO

The Food Fortress

*"for the weapons of our warfare are not of
the flesh, but divinely powerful for the
destruction of fortresses."*
(2 Cor. 10:4 NASV)

 The great evangelist, Charles Finney frequently
spoke on the subject of Satan. On one occasion,
when the service was over, a man approached
him:

"Mr. Finney, I don't believe in the devil."

The evangelist studied him thoughtfully for a moment
then replied:

"I don't either." This took his inquirer by surprise.
While the man was trying to regain his composure,
Mr. Finney continued:

**"Now I certainly believe there is a personal devil, but
I don't believe in him. Jesus called him a liar and a
murderer, denouncing him as the father of all lies. I
wouldn't believe in someone like that, and I am glad
you don't either. But as for believing he is real, all you**

have to do is try resisting him and you'll soon change your mind."

May I assume, dear reader, that the reality of Satan is unquestioned in your mind? I know some regard him as a mere figure of speech. Others think of him as an influence. Yet he is as real as the Lord Jesus and lives to damage our fellowship with God. If you doubt that, you can satisfy yourself quickly enough by taking Mr. Finney's advice. Try resisting him. He'll respond with amazing swiftness.

HOW SATAN FITS INTO GOD'S PLAN

Ages ago the devil enjoyed an exalted position in heaven. He probably ranked second to the Lord Jesus. But the day came when he coveted God's throne and conceived a plan for taking it by force. He persuaded an army of angels to join him. His plan was to depose the Almighty and install himself as the ruler of eternity. It was a matter of ego.

The plan failed, of course. There's no way for a creature to be mightier than his creator.

What did the Lord do with the devil once the plot had failed? Dispose of him? Indeed not. God is too economy-minded for that. Now that sin had found its way into His kingdom, **WHY NOT USE IT?** And that's exactly what God did. He would never throw away anything as useful as the devil. It opened the way for a terrific program which God began immediately.

He created souls in His exact image and placed them on earth. Then He set about to USE the devil to bring forth a race of TESTED citizens. That is, He would use the devil to **TEST THEIR FREE WILLS.** Thus it was that man was placed in the position of having to choose between God and Satan. The earth became man's testing ground. Now it could be determined by actual experience whether a man would love the Lord and obey Him, or shun the Lord to become the servant of Satan. It is by this means that the future citizens of heaven are screened out of the rest of mankind.

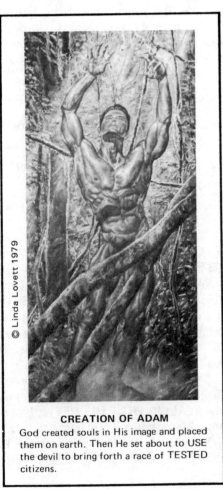

© Linda Lovett 1979

CREATION OF ADAM
God created souls in His image and placed them on earth. Then He set about to USE the devil to bring forth a race of TESTED citizens.

● For the devil to be used in this fashion, he has to be able to roam about freely as **A GOD.** This means he operates in the unseen realm of the spirit. He is a spirit. And it is perfectly proper to refer to him as the **UN-HOLY** spirit. By virtue of Adam's fall in the garden of Eden, the devil has a **LEGAL RIGHT** to approach a Christian and appeal to his old nature. Just as the Holy Spirit approaches the Christian and appeals to his new nature, so does the devil stir up the believer's carnal nature with its appetites and desires. He has been given a rather free hand when it comes to planting ideas in our minds and doing all he can, BY SUGGESTION, to weaken and hinder our spiritual growth.

Three New Testament authorities insist that:

1. Satan is the **"god of this world"** (PAUL: 2 Cor. 4:4).

2. Satan is the **"prince of this world"** (JESUS: John 14:30).

3. The whole world **"lies in the evil one"** (JOHN: 1st John 5:19).

NOTE. While the devil is given a free hand with our thought-life, he is NOT allowed to tempt us beyond our ability to cope with the temptation. The Lord knows our limitations better than we do. He holds Satan back from laying on us more than we can bear. That's a promise we can count on (I Cor. 10:13). Beyond that we're told to RESIST him and he will FLEE from us. That's also a promise (James 4:7). But reading promises in the Bible and being able to implement them into our lives are two different things. That takes know-how. It was for this reason that I wrote **DEALING WITH THE DEVIL.** I'll be mentioning this book later, because it is so important to know our enemy. It's a lot easier to resist the temptation to EAT when you know how to deal with the one TEMPTING YOU to do it.

IF YOU WERE IN SATAN'S SHOES

Satan is angry. You'd feel the same way if you were in

34

his shoes. He lost his one big chance when Jesus refused every one of his tempting offers, resisting him all the way to Calvary. Once the Lord accomplished His mission on the cross, Satan's doom was sealed. He hates Jesus for robbing him of his last chance for survival. Ever since, he has devoted himself to striking back at the Lord. But how can he do that? The Lord is beyond his reach. Yes, but there's another way he can hurt the Lord—**by damaging His children.** When a child of God is abused by the devil, it pains our precious Savior greatly.

So the devil devotes himself to doing everything he can to keep Christians from growing in the likeness of the Lord. He knows they have only this one life to get ready for the next one. If he can keep their characters and personalities from maturing in the likeness of the Lord, the **DAMAGE WILL BE ETERNAL.** The conditions necessary for changing into the Lord's likeness **DO NOT exist in heaven.** There will be NO changes after death. If a person is going to grow, he must do it on earth. **There will be NO CHANGING in heaven.** That is the nature of things eternal—they do not change. Anything that changes has to be temporal. The only way Satan can get even with the Lord, is to use his powers and advantages to keep people from coming to Christ, and after that, to keep them from maturing once they are saved.

SATAN'S EDGE

If the devil has the power to make us EAT, it will help to know **HOW** he does it. To understand his advantage, we should consider three features of his operation.

❶ Satan operates in the realm of our thoughts.

If the devil were confined to a body, as we are, he'd be limited to the five senses, able to be in only ONE PLACE AT A TIME. Beyond that, he'd also be limited TO THE BRAIN that came with his body. That is a severe limitation as we all know from experience. Operating as an UNSEEN SPIRIT, he is free of both body and brain. **Operating as a MIND, he can be in more than one place at a time.** Because he operates in the spirit, he is able to view our thoughts. Thoughts are spirit. No one can see a thought with physical eyes. **But the devil can see everything WE THINK AND FEEL.** This is why he is so familiar with our weaknesses. This is why he knows the right moment to drop a tempting idea into our thinking.

As he watches our thought-life, he follows the thought sequence as the different scenes pass before our imaginations. He can spot the ideal moment for inserting one of HIS ideas. He has to be careful. He can't be obvious about it. We'd get suspicious. His success depends on our accepting his idea **as our own.** If he got clumsy or careless, he would give himself away . . . and a person might then realize the idea wasn't his own. But with thousands of years of experience, he rarely slips up.

● Consider what this means in terms of getting us to eat when we shouldn't. We can be moving along in our routine, not thinking of food at all, when suddenly the idea occurs to us.

Suppose you've had a hard day at the job. You're on the way home. You find yourself thinking about the fine dinner your wife has waiting for you. You even see yourself sitting down to the table. There's nothing about this mental scene to make you connect it with the devil in any way. But as you think about it, you become more hungry by the mile. By the time you get home and walk in the door, you blurt out . . . , "Man, I'm starved! I could eat a horse!"

Now that's a lie. The devil's lie. You're not starving. Your body is under no real stress. You've got more fuel on board than you can use. It's just an IDEA . . . an idea linked to appetite, not to what your body needs. The idea of being starved didn't originate with your stomach. It came from your MIND. **It was SATAN'S IDEA.** How do we know? A healthy body doesn't begin to starve until it has gone for about 40 days without food. There are cases of record where obese individuals have gone as long as EIGHT MONTHS without any food at all.

NO FOOD. A classic story used by many who write about the body's need for little food, is that of Ralph Flores, a 42 year old pilot from California and 21 year old Helen Klaben, a coed from Brooklyn. While on a flight over Northern British Columbia in the dead of winter, their plane crashed into the side of a mountain. In March of 1963 the newspapers told the amazing story of how they managed to survive seven weeks in the wilderness without any food. During this time they lived on a diet of melted snow. Not only did they emerge from their ordeal in good condition, but they were also healed of their injuries suffered in the crash of their plane. I'll be speaking of them again in a later chapter, but I mention their story here to show that **missing a few meals has nothing to do with starvation.** That's the devil's idea. The stomach might growl, but not out of starvation. It's used to being filled regularly. Very clearly the starving idea and compulsion to eat ravenously comes from Satan. It is an IDEA he has dropped into your mind.

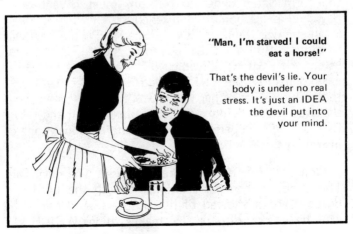

"Man, I'm starved! I could eat a horse!"

That's the devil's lie. Your body is under no real stress. It's just an IDEA the devil put into your mind.

❷ SATAN works with suggestions only.

It is important to see that Satan cannot FORCE us to eat. Because he drops an idea into our minds, it doesn't mean we have to act on it. We don't. We can reject it. Nowhere is it hinted in the Word of God that we MUST give in to the devil. **If we give in, it is because we HAVE CHOSEN to do so.** And that's the way the devil wants it. He is pleased to have us do this of our OWN FREE WILL. That way **we're** to blame. When the TV comic says, "The devil made me do it," he's misinformed. The devil can't make us do anything.

But Satan is clever. His suggestions are so subtle and disguised that he can take things which WE KNOW to be wrong, and make them appear to be right. Now that takes skill, but he's got it. It was in just this way that he got Eve to disobey God's explicit command.

You know the Eve story. God made available to Adam and Eve all the fruit of the garden. But in the middle of the garden was one tree from which they were forbidden to eat. They were content to do God's will until the day Satan approached Eve disguised as a serpent. A talking serpent (if that was indeed the form Satan chose to put on) must have been a powerful attraction. Eve listened to the devil's ideas. Soon she was thinking his way. She KNEW the fruit was forbidden. But when she looked at the tree again, **after listening to Satan,** it seemed different. Not only did it look delicious, but she believed it would benefit her; that it would make her wiser. So deceived was she, that she was ready to defy God's explicit command. Now that is a tricky operation . . . and **Satan has lost none of his touch** since.

Well the fruit didn't make her wiser. The devil lied. The action ruined her relationship with the Lord and brought about the fall of her husband. And that's the way he works with us. He makes things WHICH WE

KNOW are bad for us somehow to appear right. And he does it entirely with suggestions, just as he did with Eve. When it comes to food, he makes us think the more we eat the more satisfied we'll be. He even deceives us into eating on the basis of TASTE, rather than what is good for our bodies. As a result we consume **unhealthy** food and lots of it . . . just because we believe the devil's lie. We end up fat and dissatisfied, yet ready to eat more.

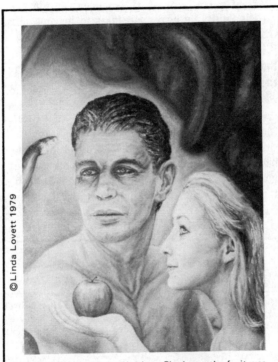

© Linda Lovett 1979

Eve listened to the devil's ideas. She knew the fruit was forbidden. But when she looked at the tree again, **after listening to Satan,** she believed it would benefit her.

❸ Satan has a perfect disguise for his operations.

Can you guess what it is? Stand in front of a mirror and you'll see it.

"Hey, wait a minute! All I see is myself!" Exactly. That's the disguise. He disguises himself **AS YOU.** He has to do this. We wouldn't have anything to do with him if he came to us **as the devil,** would we? There is no way he can approach a Christian openly. He has to be content with getting us to accept his ideas **AS OUR OWN.** When we act on them, they appear as our ideas. In this way he disguises himself as us.

> **NOTE.** The Lord Jesus does the same thing. He comes to us via His Spirit. He wants His ideas to become ours. When that happens we call the process, **"inspiration."** Scripturally it is described as . . . "Let this mind be in you," or having the mind of Christ. If we accept Jesus' ideas as our own, then HIS ideas direct our behavior. Similarly, the devil wants us to accept his ideas also. When that occurs, we call the process, **"temptation."** When we accept Satan's ideas, then his suggestions affect our behavior. Please see, though, the ONLY WAY Satan or the Lord can influence our behavior is **when we accept their ideas as our own.** It should not surprise us that the Lord and the devil both work in the same way. Both are gods, and the devil is a master counterfeiter.

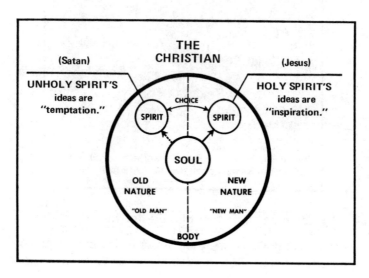

THE MIND IS THE BATTLEFIELD

The warfare in which we are involved with Satan is wholly **MENTAL:**

 "For the weapons of our warfare are not of the flesh, but divinely powerful for the destruction of fortresses. We are destroying speculations and every lofty thing raised up against the knowledge of God, and we are taking every thought captive to the obedience of Christ!" (2 Cor. 10:4,5, NASV).

During the times you have read those verses, did it ever occur to you that the apostle was describing the mind as a BATTLEFIELD? When he speaks of weapons, that's WAR TALK. He speaks of destroying fortresses and pulling down strongholds. Whose fortresses? Satan's. "Do you mean, Brother Lovett, that the devil actually builds strongholds in our minds?" That's exactly what I mean. To us they may seem like the habits or weaknesses. In reality, however, they are strongholds erected in our thought-life.

In one man's mind there might be a sex stronghold. In another liquor. Again it might be pride or the love of money. The one we're interested in right now, of course, is the stronghold of FOOD. How does Satan build such a stronghold? Easily. Working as an unseen spirit, he drops ideas into our minds. As this goes on year after year, we become **conditioned.** In time, he can get us to eat with almost no effort on his part. He then has a stronghold. After that all he has to do is sit back in his stronghold and treat us like dogs. He says, "Speak! Speak!" And we say, . . . "Food . . . Food . . . Food!"

NOTE. Consider the spiritual giant who is steadfast in prayer, who begins his day in the Word of God and looks to God to guide him all day long. He knows he must watch out for Satan. The Word tells him to. So he makes sure no evil thoughts are allowed to roost in his imagination. He refrains from judging others and he is careful not to let his eyes or ears behold anything unclean. He wants his life regulated by the Word of God. But there is one time when his guard is down . . . at mealtime. This man of God never suspects that anything as good as food could be a tool of the devil. So he eats, totally unaware that Satan is getting to him. Here's a giant of a Christian, so spiritual he can't be tempted with any gross sin, yet easy prey before a knife and fork. Now that's subtle. Very clearly the devil is using food to victimize a host of Christians whom he couldn't enslave any other way.

● If you watch for them, you'll find there are times in your routines when you are especially vulnerable to satanic food suggestions. The devil knows how to make the most of those moments. Maybe it is whenever you are alone. Or . . .

★ Doing housework

★ Watching TV

★ Listening to stereo

★ Writing letters

★ Visiting friends

★ When all the food is paid for

★ Putting away food after shopping

★ Coffee breaks

★ Coping with a crisis

★ Entertaining friends

★ Worrying

★ Fixing meals

The list is practically endless.

When something becomes a habit, it requires almost NO conscious effort.

AWARENESS. We usually put our coats on the same way, right? That is, we always shove the same arm through the sleeve. Try doing it the OPPOSITE way. I mean it, try it. It will feel most strange. Why? You are more aware of what you're doing. You suddenly notice the texture of the sleeve.

You're conscious of the effort it takes. You're aware of every movement of your arm. But when you put that coat on in the usual way, you scarcely notice what you're doing. It's a perfunctory act. You can even do it without being aware of it.

How true this is when it comes to eating. We can consume a piece of pie or a handful of nuts without **any awareness** of what we're doing. It can be as automatic as putting on a coat or shaking hands. When we do this upon Satan's suggestion, **he has a FOOD STRONGHOLD established in our minds.** When we can eat and not even remember what we've eaten, the devil is operating out of his mighty stronghold.

Satan began building this fortress in your youth. It has been going on for years. It often starts with the parental admonition . . . "Now you clean your plate. People are starving all over the world." Little by little, that stronghold becomes established.

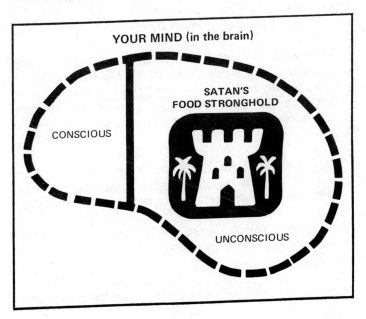

• These fortresses have to be conquered. They have to be pulled down. How did the apostle say we should do this? By bringing "thoughts into captivity." That is, gaining control over thoughts. These fortresses are built on IDEAS. They can be destroyed as we gain control over the ideas we permit in our thinking. We can tear down a stronghold by learning to REFUSE the very ideas of which it is made.

IF IT WEREN'T FOR THE DEVIL

There are few animals that will eat more than they need for sustenance. Most will eat what is right for them and STOP. How often have you seen a cow that was fatter than the rest of the herd? A sea gull too fat to fly? Or an obese giraffe? Animals in the wild, left to their natural eating patterns, rarely get fat. But how different it is with man. He eats when he is **NOT** hungry; drinks when he's **NOT** thirsty. Why? Satan has built a stronghold in his mind. All the devil has to do is whisper (ever so faintly at that) . . . "Wouldn't a little snack go good right now?" We seize that suggestion and say . . . "Man, I could sure go for a little snack right now!"

Then what? We head for the cupboard or refrigerator without realizing we're **OBEYING THE DEVIL**. From his stronghold he sits back and beams. Completely unaware that the devil is manipulating us, we consume food we don't need; food which will end up as ugly fat somewhere on our bodies.

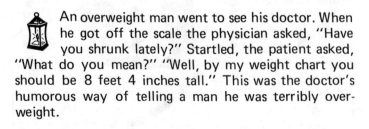 An overweight man went to see his doctor. When he got off the scale the physician asked, "Have you shrunk lately?" Startled, the patient asked, "What do you mean?" "Well, by my weight chart you should be 8 feet 4 inches tall." This was the doctor's humorous way of telling a man he was terribly overweight.

• I'm thinking of some of the popular books which

44

suggest that . . . *CALORIES DON'T COUNT.* Satan must have inspired that idea. The hard fact is, while we may not care to count calories, our bodies never forget a single one. Every calorie that goes into our mouths registers some place in the body. When 3500 of those rascals pass through our mouths, we've just put on another pound. And to think Satan starts this whole process with just one extra bite.

> **NOTE.** If the devil can get us to eat but ONE EXTRA COOKIE a day for 140 days (less than 5 months), we would have 3500 calories stored up in the form of FAT. That is 16 ounces of fat we would not have had if we laid off the cookies. Our bodies are perfect record keepers. The counting system never forgets a single calorie. I hope you'll keep that in mind when we're talking about the AMOUNTS of food we eat in later chapters.

What does this tell us? If we're going to gain control over our eating, one thing is sure—we've got to do something about the devil, and his ideas. We've got to learn HOW to catch him in the act as he tries to plant ideas in our minds. After that, we need to know how to resist him and his ideas. That's what we're going to see—next!

SUMMARY

The Lord did NOT destroy Satan after his revolt was put down. Instead, the Lord is using him to bring forth a tested race. Satan is allowed to attack us through our old natures. It is God's intention that we should resist the devil's attacks and come to maturity as a result.

ONE of the devil's ways to damage Christians is by getting them to overeat. He knows if they take ONE BITE more than they need, they are living to eat, rather than eating to live. He starts when a person is young, conditioning him to eat more than he should. As the Christian responds to Satan's suggestion, a FOOD STRONGHOLD is erected in his mind. With the passing of time, this stronghold becomes so formidable that Satan controls the believer's eating habits without his realizing it.

Since the fortress is built upon suggestions and ideas, the believer can destroy the FOOD STRONGHOLD by learning to recognize Satan's suggestions and deal with them. **If IDEAS build the fortress, then resisting those ideas can destroy it.** Complete victory in the area of overeating cannot be attained without a knowledge of the way Satan operates and a plan for resisting his attacks.

That's why **STEP ONE** in our plan has to include **instructions for dealing with the devil.**

CHAPTER THREE

Satan's Suggestions— Fiery Darts!

"Above all taking the shield of faith, wherewith ye shall be able to quench all the fiery darts of the wicked."
(Eph. 6:16 KJV)

 If you had gasoline stored in your backyard, or you kept gunpowder in a shed, would you allow youngsters with matches to get anywhere near it? Indeed you wouldn't! You'd take every precaution to see that no flame of any kind came close to that explosive material.

Well, you and I have kegs of gunpowder stored in our old natures. They are our passions, cravings, and desires. It should make us nervous to think that Satan has a quiver of "fiery darts." The apostle Paul is thinking that when he says . . .

"Above all taking the shield of faith, wherewith ye shall be able to quench all the fiery darts of the wicked" (Eph. 6:16).

● We've already seen how the devil's chief sport is making fools of God's people by using their weaknesses

47

against them. Now think of him as looking for the right moment to fire one of his flaming ideas into our gunpowder appetites. And when he does—POW! It triggers within us an impulse we can't control.

Henry Ward Beecher said . . .

"It is in our own bosom that the POWER of temptation is found. Temptation is but a spark. If it falls on ice or snow, what harm is done. None. But if it falls on gunpowder . . . watch out!"

● The gunpowder idea is but another way of picturing Satan's stronghold in our minds. The more we develop a craving for something of the flesh, the more explosive becomes our passion. As this goes on over the years, our resistance is lowered. Then all the devil has to do is drop in **one** of his flaming ideas and the power of exploding passion consumes us. Then we find ourselves driven by an overpowering impulse to please the flesh.

One of those gunpowder kegs is labeled—FOOD!

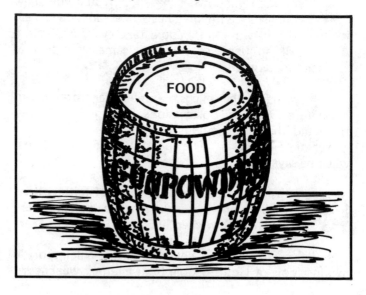

If Satan can get one of his fiery suggestions to that keg, the desire to eat will explode inside us. Now that "dart" may be nothing more than a whispered . . . "How about another spoonful of potatoes and gravy?" All it takes is a spark. Next thing you know you're saying, "Yeah, that'd be fine." And you're eating more than you need.

WE'VE GOT TO WARD OFF THOSE DARTS

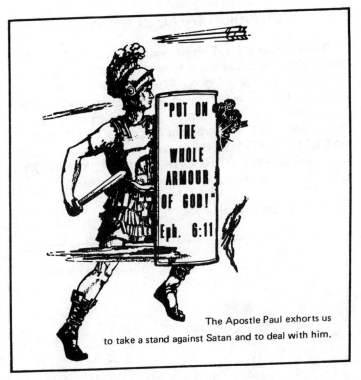

"PUT ON THE WHOLE ARMOUR OF GOD!" Eph. 6:11

The Apostle Paul exhorts us to take a stand against Satan and to deal with him.

Visualize a Roman soldier in combat. See him decked out in his armor. He carries a heavy shield on his left arm, a sword in his right hand. But take another look at that shield. The surface of it is covered with leather which has been splashed with water. That way it won't catch fire when raised to ward off a flaming arrow.

The apostle Paul employs the figure of a Roman soldier to picture the Christian's warfare with the devil (Eph. 6:10-16). How fast would a soldier have to swing his shield to intercept a dart coming his way? Well that's how fast the believer has to act to keep Satan's flaming ideas from triggering an explosion in his old nature. When it comes to intercepting the devil's darts, we don't have much time. We've got to raise the "shield of faith" in a hurry.

CATCHING SATAN IN THE ACT

Recognizing a **food attack** isn't too hard. If you feel the IMPULSE to eat something other than at meal time, or MORE THAN YOU NEED while at the table, you know the devil is behind it. But recognizing the first idea is the trick. You can do that by setting a trap for him. When you set a trap for Satan, DO NOT look for an OUTSIDE FORCE. Satan doesn't work that way. The idea will arrive **AS THOUGH IT WERE YOUR OWN.** The first notion will be an appetizing thought.

Let's watch it work.

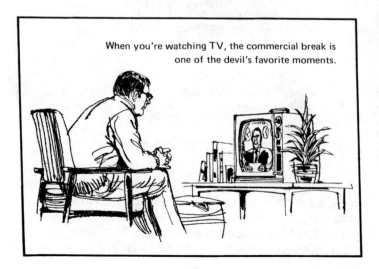

When you're watching TV, the commercial break is one of the devil's favorite moments.

You're watching TV. A commercial break is coming up. That's one of the devil's favorite moments. He actually conditions people to head for the kitchen whenever a station break occurs. But you know this now. So start watching. See if you can detect the FIRST FOOD IDEA as it arrives in your mind. You will if you're watching for it. When you do, you'll be amazed at Satan's subtlety.

THEN IT COMES. But you detect it right away—because you were expecting it.

Satan expects you to rise from your chair and head for the kitchen. But you don't. Instead you do something that startles the daylight out of him.

• **GET SET.** I'm going to ask you to do something you may have never done before—**speak aloud to the devil.** That's right, I'm going to ask you to talk to him directly.

NO DANGER. Don't be shaken by that idea. There's nothing unusual about it. You may think to yourself, "I could never address the devil directly! After all, he's the god of this world!" Oh, yes you can. When you pray, you address the God of Glory, the eternal Creator—and you do it all the time. You aren't afraid of talking to Jesus. So, if you can speak to the Lord, you can speak to the devil. Naturally, if you've never done it before, it will seem spooky the first time. But don't be afraid. He can't hurt you. Remember: his power is limited to dropping ideas into your mind. There's nothing to fear. Thousands of Christians do this many times a day and will tell you "There's nothing to it."

• How does a person talk to the devil? Just like he talks to Jesus. You picture Satan in your mind, much as you picture the Lord in your imagination. That's the purpose of the imagination—to give reality to unseen things. Jesus is real, so is Satan. Since we're limited to

51

the finite things of this world, God has equipped us with this amazing ability called imagination. With it we can picture unseen things. You don't have to visualize a detailed form. Whatever comes to mind when you think of the devil will do nicely. If it's just a shadowy presence, that is OK. You can speak to that. It isn't necessary to conjure a vivid image of the devil. No matter what form he takes in your "mind's eye" (imagination), speak to him something like this . . .

ACTION

You're still seated on the sofa. Don't get up. Close your eyes if you wish. That usually helps when addressing someone in your imagination. Very quickly now . . .

"Satan, in the name of Jesus go away. I know what you're up to, but I don't need any food. Take your suggestion and get away from me, for it is written . . . My 'body is the temple of the Holy Spirit.' "

Wow! Does that catch him by surprise! He's stunned.

Are those exact words necessary? No. Any words spoken with authority will do. But they must be addressed to Satan directly. You have to speak to him. You can't deal with the devil by talking to God in prayer. Satan is never bothered by that.

DIRECTLY. Some Christians have strange notions about dealing with Satan. A story circulated among believers tells about a young lady who was asked if it bothered her when the devil tempted her to do evil. "Yes," she replied, "but when the devil knocks at the door of my will, I just say . . . 'Lord Jesus, will you please answer the door!' Then when Satan sees the Lord he runs away." You've heard the story. It has a cute sound to it, but it just doesn't work that way. The Lord's presence in our lives does not keep Satan from attacking us. There's no way to get the Lord to do what He

52

has clearly told us to do. **"Resist the devil and he will flee from you!"** Some feel we enjoy automatic protection from Satan because our indwelling Lord is greater than he. It just isn't so. It is the Lord's plan for us to meet Satan's attacks and resist them. This is how we are to grow strong. The presence of Christ **in us guarantees** that we **CAN DEAL** with Satan and put him to flight **IF WE WANT TO.** But there's **nothing automatic about it.** For us to be victorious, we have to face him in combat and win!

● So talking to God about the devil has no effect. The Lord **WANTS US** to stand up to him and **TAKE AUTHORITY** OVER HIM. Remember: we are not begging Satan to go, we're not asking him to go. **We're COMMANDING him to depart,** just as Jesus did in the wilderness temptation (Matt. 4:1-11). There are no specific words to say. You could even put the command like this . . .

"Go away Satan, I'll have nothing to do with your ideas. The Lord Jesus is my Master. In His name I command you to depart for it is written . . . 'Whatsoever you do in word or deed, do all in the name of the Lord Jesus . . . !' He is the One Who leads my life, not you!"

THEN WHAT?

Satan goes. He has to. You have the authority. The only qualification is—**you MUST MEAN what you say.** If you don't really mean the command, the devil won't go. And since he can read your thoughts, he knows when you truly mean something and when you don't. Sometimes he knows it better than you do. He's very sharp when it comes to understanding people's motives.

When Satan goes you feel it. There is an immediate release. The pressure subsides. The urge to eat passes. It is thrilling to experience that release. But here's something you should know. That release can last for only a few moments . . . or as long as your guard is up. Why? As soon as you forget about Satan, allowing your mind to become busy with something else, he'll slip back. He waits for another unsuspecting moment, ready to insert another EAT idea. So you have to WATCH.

• Does the word "watch" remind you of something? The Lord Jesus said, **"WATCH and pray, lest ye enter into temptation"** (Mark 14:38). What comes first in that exhortation? WATCHING! We're to watch for Satan even before we pray. Why? The devil can get to us even when we're praying. Anytime you're engaged in a military operation, and we are, the key word is WATCH.

> **HINT.** The instant Satan departs (which is immediately upon your command), turn your mind to the Lord. The TV commercials are still going on. During that time, thank the Lord for giving you authority to deal with the devil and for backing your command with such power. Praise Him for teaching you how to defend yourself against such a persistent enemy. Let your mind go to the day when you will be reigning with Jesus in His kingdom. Praise Him that He is teaching you how to handle authority NOW. Your heart will probably be pounding. If this is the first time you have experienced the flight of Satan on your command, you'll be flush with victory. The commercials are over. So back to your program.

WHAT IS SATAN DOING?

He's lurking somewhere in the shadows of your old nature. He left the battlefield, but he hasn't gone far. There's no telling when he'll try again. He doesn't play the game by any rules except his own. He may not bother you again all evening, or he might come back with the next set of commercials. The thing to do is remain alert. A Roman sentry was executed, you know, when he was found asleep at his post. So don't let your guard down.

You know he'll be back with **another FOOD SUGGES-TION**—you just don't know when.

● When Satan returns with another food idea, be ready to do the same thing again. Be prepared to make a **"quick draw"** and command him to go . . .

"I know you're trying to dominate me with food, Satan. So in the name of Jesus Go . . . get off my back! The Bible says 'Delight thyself in the Lord and He will give thee the desires of thine heart.' I have set my heart on Christ . . . so take off!"

You see it doesn't really matter what you say to the devil as long as you **COMMAND** him to depart in the name of the Lord, and back it up with the Word of God. He is not afraid of us, but **when we stand against him IN CHRIST**, it is another matter. He has to go . . . for he is a **defeated** enemy. Defeated by the Lord, that is. And when you quote the Word, it is like a SWORD THRUST to his soul. In fact, it is only when the Word is used in this fashion that it becomes the **"sword of the Spirit"** (Eph. 6:17). The way you word your command is im-material.

Do this every time Satan returns. If he assaults you 20 times in the same evening, resist him 20 times. It is a bat-tle, I won't deceive you about that. Paul speaks of it as "wrestling." But here's some helpful insight: Satan has a HUGE EGO. He hates being rejected. Every time you order him away, he suffers fierce pain. Without doubt, you can keep it up a lot longer than he can take it. For you, this is FUN in the Spirit. You actually rejoice as the power of the Spirit becomes yours. While he, on the other hand, is **BRUISED** every time you order him away.

The devil will try you. That is, he'll test you to see if you really mean business. He wants to know if you'll give up before he will. That's why he might come back 20 or 30 times in a single evening. As soon as he is convinced you're not about to give in, he'll depart and leave you alone for quite a spell. But even that is tricky. He knows that if he gives you an extended rest from his assaults, you might drop your guard. Then he'll be back in a flash. **His withdrawals are ALWAYS STRATEGIC.** His eyes are never off of you for a second. Like our eternal God Who, "neither slumbers nor sleeps," so does the devil keep a watchful eye on our souls. He's like a hungry lioness, stalking a gazelle.

> **NOTE.** What I have given you in this chapter and the one before it, has been a skimpy explanation of the way Satan works and how to deal with him. The full particulars of his operation and how to set up your own defense system are found in my book, **DEALING WITH THE DEVIL.** However, I have given you enough information to resist his food suggestions. You owe it to yourself to learn as much as you can about Satan and how to defend yourself against him. There are other areas of your life where you may be **even more** susceptible to his attacks than in the matter of food. I hope you'll take my advice and make this book a part of your arsenal. It really is great to be able to break the devil's power and pull down one stronghold after another. I guarantee this book will do as much to change your life as anything you can read. **I'm asking God to let me put a copy in every Christian home.**

WHAT WE'VE ACCOMPLISHED SO FAR

We have discussed Satan's fiery darts (suggestions) and how they can ignite our gunpowder appetites. He can trigger the impulse to eat by dropping a single FOOD idea into our thought-life. We don't suspect Satan's part in it, because it appears **as our own idea.** We have learned (in brief, to be sure) how to recognize Satan's suggestion and head it off before it ignites our passion for food.

Why is it necessary to do this? We need breathing room so we can go to work on DEFUSING THE DYNAMITE in our old natures. There is no way to go into the devil's territory and pull down one of his STRONGHOLDS without first binding him. That is, **we have to keep Satan off our backs while we demolish the FOOD STRONGHOLD.** By keeping him at bay, as I have described in this chapter, we have a free hand to do that. But as long as he DOMINATES our appetite, we're in no position to attack his fortress. Now praise God, we can resist him and give ourselves that opportunity. When you behold the remarkable way God has provided for us to PULL DOWN the food stronghold, you're going to be thrilled. That's next.

WE HAVE COMPLETED THE FIRST PHASE OF OUR THREE STEP PLAN FOR GETTING THE WEIGHT OFF AND KEEPING IT OFF.

I TRUST YOU SEE HOW NECESSARY IT IS TO BE ABLE TO DEAL WITH THE DEVIL BEFORE WE TRY DEALING WITH OUR BODIES.

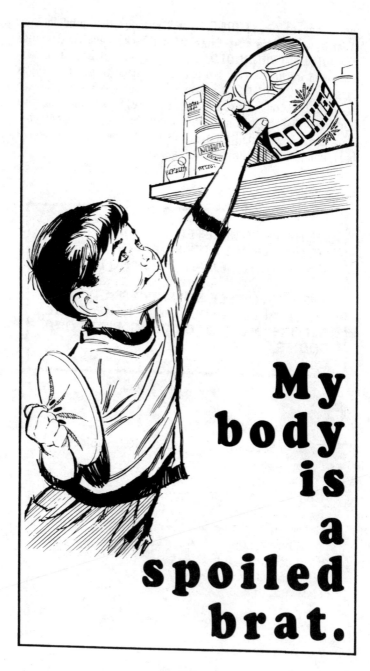

My body is a spoiled brat.

PHASE TWO

How to gain control over your body

This is one of the most vital subjects a Christian can consider. Yet my approach to it might startle you. You can be sure of this— God has blessed this approach for centuries. In recent times, this God-given practice has fallen into disuse. But you're about to re-discover it. Again, I ask you to keep in mind that the most important part of this book is PHASE THREE. So stay with me. Don't let a minor truth keep you from the big one.

CHAPTER FOUR

Pulling Down Satan's Food Stronghold

*"I beseech you therefore, brethern, by the
mercies of God that ye present your
bodies a living sacrifice, holy, acceptable
unto God, which is your reasonable service."*
(Rom. 12:1 KJV)

A bit of farmer wisdom says you can't kill a frog by dropping him in boiling water. He reacts so quickly to the sudden heat, he leaps out before he's hurt. But if you put him in cold water and gradually warm it, he never decides to jump until it's too late. By then he's cooked.

That's the way the devil eases us into food addiction. We don't realize we're in trouble with our eating habits until it's too late. We don't suspect anything is wrong until those unsightly pounds appear. By then, of course, it's too late. We have already developed such a passion for food, we no longer have the will to eat only what we need. At that point we're cooked.

● Without our realizing it the devil has constructed a **FOOD STRONGHOLD** in our minds.

SUCH A TINY SIN TOO

Most of us shy away from big sins. We shudder at the thought of being caught in a big sin that could wipe out our testimony. So we guard against drunkenness, immorality, stealing and violence. It would be awful to bring shame on the Lord and ourselves. Yet we make no defense against the little sins. Often, that's the kind the devil uses to penetrate our wills.

When a business corporation erects a new building it is greatly concerned with earthquakes and fire protection. It fears a calamity that would ruin everything. But if that same corporation were constructing a wharf in Central America, it's prime concern would be for tiny creatures in the water known as Teredos. These creatures, so small they can be seen only with a microscope, immediately begin boring their way through the piling under water. They make no noise. Before long, though, if a person were to push against one of those pilings, it would topple as if cut by a saw.

Food is so innocent. A wee bit of overeating is like a Teredo. The evil seems so tiny. That's why Christians take it to their bosom. Yet it is all the devil needs for a small penetration. A few little Teredos (extra bites) on the job and our wills **crumble** in time.

SATAN MUST WORK IN THIS FASHION

God has made our wills sovereign. That is, we **don't** have to do anything we don't WANT TO. The human will is a mighty citadel, an impregnable castle. There is no way Satan can conquer it from the outside. He can try storming the walls and crashing the gate, but it won't do him any good. There is no way for him to charge through and overpower our wills. There's no way he can make ANY penetration without OUR COOPER-

ATION. The gate to the castle of our wills **has to be OPENED FROM THE INSIDE.**

Who'd suspect FOOD to be one of the devil's CHIEF TOOLS for penetrating our wills? It's so subtle. It might take him years to actually accomplish the penetration, but he's in no hurry. Little by little he gets us to eat more than we need, and when we do he's expanded his influence by that much. Without our realizing it, we open the gate to him. After years of working silently and carefully like this, he ends up with a pretty good hold on our wills. **Then the day comes when we find our APPE-TITE is stronger than our wills.** When that happens, the devil has his fortress. Imagine—a **FOOD FORTRESS** built in our own minds!

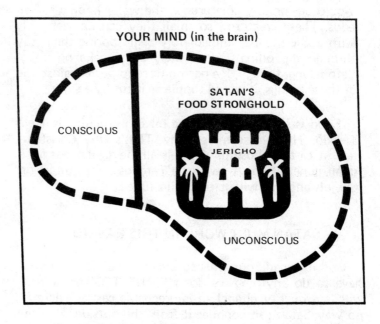

YOUR MIND (in the brain)

SATAN'S
FOOD STRONGHOLD

CONSCIOUS

JERICHO

UNCONSCIOUS

● Once that fortress is set up and in operation, Satan can make us eat EXTRA FOOD with the slightest nudge. Why, just the odor from a donut shop or bakery could be enough to make us indulge. Or again, it might be the sight of a dish of mixed nuts on the table. The point is: after he's gained his foothold, it's surprising how easily we obey HIS whims when it comes to food.

That fortress has to come down.

TEARING DOWN THE FOOD STRONGHOLD

When the children of Israel entered the promised land, the mighty fortress of Jericho stood squarely in their path. They didn't dare go around it. It would be dangerous to leave such a formidable bastion behind them. They'd never enjoy peace in the land if that great stronghold were allowed to remain. But how would they do it? Coming off the desert, they had no engines of war with which to besiege the city. Somehow those walls had to come down. Well, they did, as you know. For the Israelites carried out God's instructions for taking the city. They marched around the city for six days. On the seventh day they blew their trumpets and the walls came tumbling down.

Well the devil's FOOD STRONGHOLD in our minds is our Jericho. It's squarely in the path of our Christian progress. We can't go around it any more than the Israelites could go around their Jericho. To do so would leave the devil with a permanent foothold on our wills. We'd be under his influence for the rest of our lives. Besides, he would be able to expand his influence to one area after another as our weaknesses fell prey to his fiery darts. No, there's no alternative—that stronghold has to come down.

NOTE. You know the story of the conquest of Jericho. You know the outlandish method God used to bring down those walls. Well, what I am going to suggest for you in this chapter, may seem just as unbelievable. But if you ask the Holy Spirit about it, and get His witness, you won't care how strange the method seems . . . you'll do it. When the Lord backs something, it can't miss. Just as those Jericho walls

63

came tumbling down, so will the walls of the devil's food fortress. You may feel a little astonished at what I am going to ask you to do, so you might as well get ready to discuss it with the Lord. If you thought Satan got upset with what you encountered in Chapter One, wait until you see the fight he puts up when you get ready to carry out what I have in mind for you in this chapter.

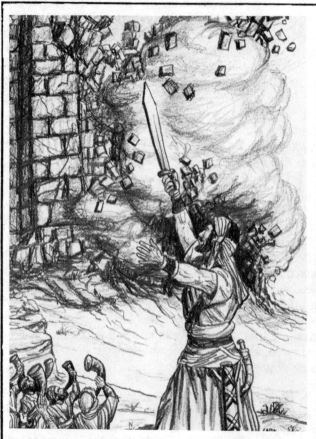

The devil's **food stronghold** in our minds is our Jericho. It's squarely in the path of our Christian progress. We can't go around it any more than the Israelites could go around their Jericho. As with the Israelites' Jericho, ours must come down too.

• It's distressing to think of the devil as having a fortress in your mind. It's not an easy fact to face. But it's true. ALL you have to do is grab hold of some of that ugly fat around your middle, and you'll have to agree your eating habits are **beyond YOUR control.** Someone else is in control. Can you see the devil's work in the things you eat? You like so many things which are really BAD for your body . . . things like candy and cokes, donuts and desserts. When you tear down Satan's stronghold, those things will go out of your life. When they do, it will be **PROOF** that you're back in command of your own eating habits.

Is your body going to let you give up these things easily? Is your appetite going to let you take over without a struggle? Not if Satan can help it. You're in for a FIGHT, my friend. But what do you expect when you tackle an enemy stronghold? Any time you try to dislodge an enemy from his base of operation you've got a WAR on your hands. Your body is going to become a real battlefield before this is over.

THINK OF IT THIS WAY

 A wise old pastor gave this advice to those of his people who could not manage their passion for food:

"TREAT YOUR BODY AS THOUGH IT WERE A SPOILED CHILD, AND IT WAS YOUR RESPONSIBILITY TO TRAIN IT."

Do you see what he means? He says you've got to be objective about your own body, as though it were separated from you. You must see it as a **SPOILED BRAT** whom God has turned over to you to train. As you listen to its cries for more meat and potatoes and gravy; more ice cream and desserts, more potato chips and pizzas, you are to treat it as a child that has been spoiled rotten. As this fussy brat presses his demands on you, you've got to get tough. Say to him . . .

"No! You've been pampered long enough. I've given in to you too many times already. We're bringing this thing to an end right now. You can beg and fuss all you want, but you're not getting another thing until you learn to eat what I say you should and no more."

● To speak to a spoiled brat with those words is a SHOCK. When you back it up with action, he knows his easy ways have come to an end. Can you guess what's coming? Your body is in for a shock. I don't mean electric shock, but something just as startling—GOING WITHOUT FOOD FOR A PERIOD OF TIME.

Yes, I'm talking about FASTING!

FASTING . . . . !

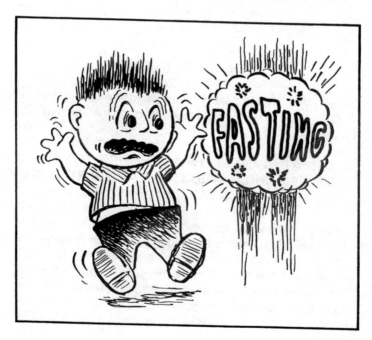

For the purpose of this book, fasting is abstaining from all foods, but continuing to drink water as needed.

Remember the TV commercials showing the bugs so terrified at the word . . . "R-A-I-D!" You probably feel something of that dread when I speak of "FASTING!" Your heart almost stops. Without my saying anything further, you know this is something you're not interested in whatsoever. Why, you'd rather try anything . . . but fasting. I can guess what Satan is doing in your mind right now. Wow! So I hasten to tell you something about fasting you may not know. It should make you feel easier about it:

WHEN A PERSON FASTS, THE CRAVING FOR FOOD LASTS FOR ABOUT 48 HOURS. AFTER THAT, HUNGER VANISHES. THE LONGING DISAPPEARS. ONCE YOU'RE OVER THE HUNGER HUMP, YOU CAN GO FOR 30 OR 40 DAYS OR MORE WITHOUT SOLID FOOD. PEOPLE HAVE FASTED FOR AS LONG AS EIGHT MONTHS WITH NO ILL EFFECTS.

Those who have no experience with fasting see it as one long fight; one long battle against hunger pains. That's not the case. Hunger vanishes in a short time. Let's turn to Matthew Four, to the place where it tells of Jesus' temptation in the wilderness, and I think you'll see something you may have missed before. Do you find the place where it says He fasted 40 days and 40 nights? Good. You're familiar with that. But have you paid attention to the next words . . . **"He THEN became hungry?"** (Vs. 2). The Lord experienced **NO HUNGER** DURING His fast. When He finally did feel hunger, it was His body's way of letting Him know the fast was over; that it was time to eat again. (Our bodies do that). That's why Satan's suggestion that He turn stones into bread was a valid temptation. He **WAS** hungry now. Yet for the past 37 or 38 days, He suffered no hunger at all.

67

There is no hunger until it's time for the body to eat again.

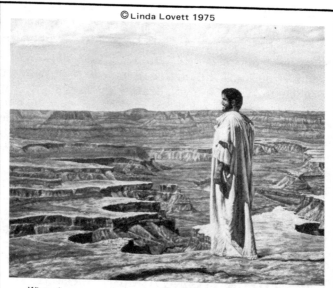
© Linda Lovett 1975

When Jesus was tempted in the wilderness, He experienced **no hunger** during His fast. When He finally did feel hunger, it was His body's way of letting Him know the fast was over.

• Don't get up tight. I'm not going to suggest anything like a 40 day fast. The spiritual victory we're after (bringing our bodies under control) can be accomplished in ten days.

NOTE. Fasting is a fabulous way to take off weight, but that's **NOT** our reason for using it. We want to **destroy Satan's stronghold** in your mind and gain control of your appetite. You WILL lose weight, as much, perhaps, as 15 to 20 pounds. The psychological effect of shedding those unwanted pounds will be most encouraging. It makes it easier to develop a new attitude toward yourself, one which says, "Hey! This is great! It's going to be fun getting myself back in shape!" Beyond that, being able to silence the cries of your flesh is going to give you a terrific boost spiritually. You'll be able to say with Paul, "I buffet my body . . . and make it my servant."

The purpose of this fast is to let your body know YOU ARE THE BOSS. The "spoiled brat" gets the message when it's impressed on him like this. It may seem like a strange way to conquer a fortress, but Satan's stronghold is so firmly established, it won't come down any other way. Forcing your body into submission through fasting, is no more strange than marching around a city and blowing trumpets. After you get a taste of what fasting can do for you, you'll agree it is **GOD'S WAY for destroying the devil's strongholds.**

The business of controlling the body and conquering our appetites, is not something I have dreamed up. The apostle Paul spoke frequently of this very thing. Again and again he urges believers to bring their bodies INTO SUBJECTION . . . even to the point of making it A SLAVE . . .

"I buffet my body and make it MY SLAVE, lest possibly, after I have preached to others, I myself should be disqualified" (I Cor. 9:27, NASV).

WHY THIS IS SO VITAL

As long as Satan has ANY control over your body whatsoever, your body is no longer yours to present to the Lord. Consider that solemn fact in the light of a verse which should be familiar to every Christian . . .

"I beseech you therefore, brethren, by the mercies of God that ye present your bodies a living sacrifice, holy, acceptable unto God, which is your reasonable service" (Rom. 12: 1).

I'm sure you've weighed that verse more than once. And deep in your heart you long to do what Paul asks. But dear friend, there is NO WAY to present to God something **which is NOT UNDER YOUR CONTROL.** There is no way to present your body to God as long as the devil retains dominion over any part of it. The plain truth is, if you're overweight, YOU CAN'T present your body to God, simply because you don't have it under your control. Those extra pounds are proof of the devil's dominion. I know that's an awful thing to face, but I'm certain the Holy Spirit is bearing witness to my words. You're not just reading another book at this point. You're facing a deep, spiritual crisis in your life.

Time was, when you were in control of your body. But now the devil, deceiving you with food, has gained dominion over your body through your appetite. He has a foothold on your will. Therefore tearing down his stronghold is not just a curious idea in a book. It is something you must regard seriously . . . and be willing to do no matter **HOW MUCH EFFORT IT TAKES.** Once you have your body under control, you can then present it to God. But until that time, you most assuredly cannot. It's not yours to present.

Opposite is a medical chart showing standard weight for given heights. You can see what your weight SHOULD BE. The difference between what you should weigh and actually do weigh, **is a measure of the devil's hold on your will.** Maybe, in your case, a more useful way of setting your goal, would be to remember how much you weighed when you were 22. That will be pretty close for most people.

YOU CAN'T AFFORD NOT TO FAST

If fasting seems impossible for you or just down-right repulsive, the alternative is worse. If you don't do something about Satan's control over your appetite, he'll

DESIRABLE WEIGHTS FOR MEN AND WOMEN AGED 25 AND OVER* in pounds according to height and frame, in indoor clothing and shoes

HEIGHT		SMALL FRAME	MEDIUM FRAME	LARGE FRAME
MEN				
FEET	INCHES			
5	4	118-126	124-136	132-148
5	5	121-129	127-139	135-152
5	6	124-133	130-143	138-156
5	7	128-137	134-147	142-161
5	8	132-141	138-152	147-166
5	9	136-145	142-156	151-170
5	10	140-150	146-160	155-174
5	11	144-154	150-165	159-179
6	0	148-158	154-170	164-184
6	1	152-162	158-175	168-189
6	2	156-167	162-180	173-194
6	3	160-171	167-185	178-199
6	4	164-175	172-190	182-204
WOMEN				
4	10	92-98	96-107	104-119
4	11	94-101	98-110	106-122
5	0	96-104	101-113	109-125
5	1	99-107	104-116	112-128
5	2	102-110	107-119	115-131
5	3	105-113	110-122	118-134
5	4	108-116	113-126	121-138
5	5	111-119	116-130	125-142
5	6	114-123	120-135	129-146
5	7	118-127	124-139	133-150
5	8	122-131	128-143	137-154
5	9	126-135	132-147	141-158
5	10	130-140	136-151	145-163
5	11	134-144	140-155	149-168

*adapted from Metropolitan Life Insurance Co., New York.

expand his influence to other areas of your life, then you'll have even less to dedicate to Jesus. You can't afford that. If you allow the devil to continue his dominion, and do so knowingly after reading this book . . . then you could find yourself covered with shame when it's your turn to meet Jesus face to face. If fasting seems rough, it is child's play compared to being "ashamed before Him at His appearing" (1st John 2:28).

• Few of us EASE into big changes in our lives. For most of us it takes a CRISIS to get us to make a dramatic change. We have to get sick, lose a child, have an accident, see a marriage go sour . . . things like that . . . before we change. **None of us changes until he HAS TO.** Well, the whole idea of fasting brings such a CRISIS . . . a needed crisis. Think of it as a crisis in your life. That's just what it is.

> **NOTE.** The devil knows the power of fasting. The idea that you would consider such a thing sends him into panic. That panic will find its way into your mind. You'll be spitting out objections to fasting in rapid fire succession . . . "It's out of the question! I could never go without food for 10 days! I'd die!" One after another of these objections will surface in your mind. It will be the devil's doing. The last thing in this world he wants you to consider is fasting. He's gained his control over your body through food . . . and here you are thinking of giving up FOOD! He knows what that will do to his control. So he will do his utmost to put the pressure on your appetite. Quite frankly, the odds are in his favor. You already have it in your mind that you must eat 2 or 3 meals a day to survive. That isn't so, but you don't know that yet. The temptation will be to HEED his suggestions.

You may have to deal with Satan even as you read these lines. The reaction he creates in your spirit could be so violent, that you will have to silence him before you can proceed. You're trying to focus on what I am saying, yet a voice in the back of your mind keeps saying . . . "I could never in this world survive a 10 day fast." What Satan wants is for you to close the book and run from the idea. He may even suggest, "Don't read any more, then you won't be responsible for the insight coming from those pages!" I trust you won't do that. But instead deal with the devil and stay with me. If you can, it'll be solid evidence you mean business in gaining control over your eating.

Talk to him like this:

"Satan, my mind is open to the Holy Spirit. He is the One Who tells me what to do. Not you. I've committed my life to Jesus and if He wants me to fast, I will. So I command you in His Name to depart from me, for it is written . . . 'present your bodies a living sacrifice unto God . . . !' "

● Did you do that? Good. With the satanic pressure removed, you'll be able to listen to the Holy Spirit. His witness will be clear now that Satan has backed off. You will be able to check what I am saying against the Spirit's witness and know whether or not I speak truly. It's the witness of the Spirit that you heed, not C. S. Lovett. Besides you should take a moment to consider the nice new weapon that has been added to your arsenal.

NEW WEAPON. Chances are you didn't know that hunger only lasts for about 48 hours after you stop eating. And the very idea of fasting meant suffering hunger pangs for days and days. That's the way most people think about it. They are surprised to learn that the hunger interval is so short . . . and even then, that the attacks of hunger last only for about 15 minutes. That's why a glass of water, which can give you a full feeling for about 15 minutes, is so effective. Get this knowledge into your thinking and fasting is a different ball game. It certainly takes a lot of the steam out of Satan's suggestions. He would like for you to believe it is something you could never do, when in reality it is something you can EASILY DO. Lay hold of this knowledge, and you have a new weapon for repelling his attacks. The reason hunger lasts for 48 hours, is because it takes that long for the body to **shift over from burning FOOD to burning FAT.** Food can last in the system for approximately 48 hours and not until it has all been consumed, does the body become a fat burner.

DOING IT WITH THE LORD

A ten day fast can be FUN—if you do it with the Lord Jesus. Is it right for a Christian to undertake any major step without first making sure it is His will? Of course not. If you were planning to leave on a trip, you'd spend time making sure you had everything you might need. Similarly, we should spend time with the Lord to make sure it is His will for us to undertake a fast and that we can count on His blessing each step of the way. So part of our preparation for fasting, is getting ready to do it WITH the Lord. He's already taught us . . . "Without Me, ye can do nothing" (John 15:5).

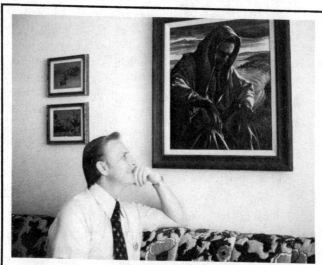

We should spend time with the Lord to make sure it is His will for us to undertake a fast and that we can count on His blessing each step of the way.

• Once you have spent time with the Lord and have His witness, you can proceed to fast with joy. It can be **FUN** to watch that SPOILED BRAT settle down as your passion for food subsides. Also, you can go into the fast **WITHOUT FEAR** of damaging your body. I know this is one of your great concerns. It is also something that Satan can be counted on to throw at you steadily. When the Lord is in it, there is no need to FEAR. You won't hurt yourself. I understand there is a natural fear which accompanies anything the first time you try it. I can tell you right now, if you can bring yourself to lean on the Lord and let Him worry about your body, you can have **FUN ON A FAST!** It can be exciting to watch the spiritual and physical changes take place.

> **NOTE.** Did you ever think of your stomach as an **ORGAN OF FAITH?** When you take no food (only water) into your system, the demands of the flesh subside allowing your spiritual appetite to rise. Not only does hunger leave, but so does your sex drive and the desire for **THINGS OF THIS WORLD.** The old nature quiets down when you fast **as unto the Lord.** You find yourself on a higher spiritual plane. What does that tell us? There's a close relationship between the body and the spirit, so close in fact, that when the stomach is empty, the heart is ready to be filled by God. On the other hand, when the stomach is full, due to overeating, you have little interest in the things of God. Your closeness to the Lord during this spiritual fast is going to be a mighty weapon for destroying the devil's power. Anytime you put the Lord ahead of food, remarkable things can occur in your soul. This is why fasting is not a strange way to bring the body into subjection after all. When you fast by faith, **that SPOILED BRAT is transformed into a delightful child;** one you're pleased with.

THE SCRIPTURAL BASIS FOR FASTING

A number of Christian authors have published books on fasting. They all build a solid case from the Scriptures. For that reason, I don't have to use a lot of space setting forth the strategic place fasting occupies in the Word of God. Actually it is so prominent, you wonder how the devil has been able to keep it under wraps. If you are interested in the way some of these writers have approached fasting from the Word of God, you'll find the works of these men helpful:

Arthur Wallis . . . . **"God's Chosen Fast"**

Franklin Hall . . . . **"Atomic Power with God"**

Derek Prince . . . . **"Shaping History Through Prayer and Fasting"**

Some excellent secular writers are:

Herbert M. Shelton . . . . . **"Fasting Can Save Your Life"**

Arnold De Vries . . . . **"Therapeutic Fasting"**

Allan Cott . . . . **"Fasting: The Ultimate Diet"**

Once you are aware that fasting really is for God's people, you suddenly see it everywhere in His Word. It is much like getting a new car. You suddenly notice all the others on the road that are like yours. They were there all the time, but you didn't have any reason to pay particular attention to them before. When you look at the great men of the Bible, you find they were devoted to prayer and fasting. All of the great accomplishments of the Bible were attended by prayer and fasting. Here are a few stars of fasting:

★ David wrote his great psalms after fasting. It was fasting that made it possible for his spirit to soar to such great heights, that he could lay hold of the wondrous revelations we find in his psalms. We have his own testimony that this is so: Psa. 35:13; 69:10; 78:18-32 and many more.

★ When Jonah declared to the people of Nineveh what God had in store for them, they believed the prophet and declared a solemn fast. The city was spared (Jonah 3:5,10).

★ When Daniel wanted to know God's will, the revelation he sought came to him via fasting (Dan. 9:3).

★ Moses took neither water nor food with him into Sinai on two separate occasions. This was a SUPERNATURAL FAST which kept the flesh completely out of the way while he communed with the Lord (Deut. 9:18; Ex. 34:28). Note this was a supernatural fast. Normally a person should never go without water for more than 3 days.

★ When the Lord was baptized in the Jordan and anointed with the Holy Spirit, he went immediately into the wilderness for a 40 day fast. This was to prepare Him for His encounter with the devil (Matt. 4:2). Remember: He was tested AS A MAN, the same as we.

★ When the apostles wanted to know God's will with regard to the first missionary journey, they gave themselves to fasting and prayer (Acts 13:2,3).

Do you have a topical Bible? You know, the kind that gathers together all the Scriptures pertaining to a certain subject. If you do, turn to the subject of fasting and see all of the Bible passages relating to it. I think you'll be impressed. You could do the same thing with a Bible concordance. When you behold all those references, you will be convinced of the importance of fasting in the Biblical program.

Those with depth in God's Word realize I could spend many pages exhausting what the Bible has to say about fasting. See—the devil has done a good job in blinding

God's people to the place fasting holds in His plan. Satan doesn't want Christians discovering the **awesome power of a spiritual fast.** In your heart you should be thankful God has used your weight problem to bring you to the place where you would consider fasting. The Lord works in strange ways. Fasting is going to be a wonderful blessing to you in gaining control over your body. That same control is going to extend to other areas of your life.

I know what's in your mind now. You would like to know just what you could expect if you were to get serious about fasting, right? That's what we're going to discuss next.

SUMMARY

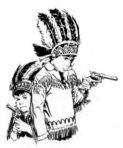

When I was a boy, we used to build play forts out of any kind of material we could get our hands on. Then we'd have mock wars. Most boys grow up learning about forts. But Satan's forts are different. They are built out of **IDEAS.** When he can get us to go for one of his ideas, he tries it again. When he is repeatedly successful with the same idea, we become CONDITIONED TO IT. We soon reach the place where we AUTOMATICALLY respond to that idea whenever he drops it in our minds. This conditioning provides the devil with his STRONGHOLD.

Therefore to pull down a Satanic stronghold, we must bring those SAME IDEAS under our control. Sound familiar? It should. This is but another way of saying . . . "bringing into captivity every thought to the obedience of Christ." Those words, of course, are part of the apostle Paul's counsel for pulling down the strongholds of Satan (2 Cor. 10:5). If a fort is made out of AN IDEA, the way to pull it down is to gain control of that idea.

78

Here's how we have approached that control so far:

1. We have learned to catch Satan in the act of dropping an idea in our minds, then ordering him away along with his idea—in the name of Jesus. This eases the pressure for a time.

2. We have also learned that part of Satan's strategy is the CONDITIONING of our bodies to respond to his FOOD IDEAS. Therefore we must DE-CONDITION OUR BODIES, so they no longer respond to his food suggestions. How do we do that? We look on our body as a SPOILED BRAT and DENY it any more food until we have regained the control. This takes about 10 days of living on water only. While a dramatic weight loss does occur, our real purpose in fasting is the regaining of the control of our bodies.

3. When we fast, the CRIES OF THE FLESH SUBSIDE. When they do, the spiritual side of our being ascends and takes over our thought-life. During the fast, we have BOTH body and thoughts under our control. In this fashion we PULL DOWN Satan's stronghold because our minds are free from Satanic pressure.

Once we have gained this control, we want to keep it. We do that by re-programming our minds with a new attitude toward food. That comes later in the book. What is important here is the connection between FOOD and spirituality. If money can come between God and man, so can food. Christians do not think of food as a spiritual problem, but when it can be said . . . "whose god is their belly," it is clear that food is more spiritual than we have suspected. The devil wants Christians to keep stuffing themselves, not only to make them fat, but to blind them to what would be theirs if they put Christ ahead of their stomachs.

Now to see what's involved when you get serious about fasting.

DOES THE IDEA OF FASTING FRIGHTEN YOU?

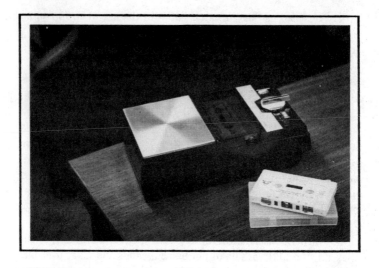

In the last chapter I tried to ease you into the idea of fasting. I hope I did a good job. If I did, you'll consider fasting without undue concern. Of course there are first time fears for anything new. You can expect those. However, if you are still not satisfied this is something the Lord wants you to do, I have prepared a special cassette that deals with fasting from the Word of God as well as discussing what happens in your body when you fast. Side one of this cassette helps you weigh the idea of going on a fast as part of this plan. You will be satisfied that it is a natural part of life, something God has provided. When you hear the spiritual benefits of fasting, I know you'll be eager to try it with the Lord.

Side two of this cassette is used after you begin your fast. It is called . . . "Getting over the hump" (No. 544). And that's just what it does. It helps you get through the hunger period. While this cassette is not needed to make this plan work in your life, it can be a big help at the hardest point — getting started and managing the hunger pains of the first 48 hours.

CHAPTER FIVE

What To Expect When You Fast

"And after He had fasted forty days and forty nights, He then became hungry."
(Matt. 4:2 NASV)

I won't forget the terror I felt one night. I had been awakened by a sound. To this day I don't know what it was. But it got me out of bed and prowling through the house to investigate. A street light streaming through the windows made it possible for me to slip about without having to turn on the house lights. As I silently moved toward my study I froze in my tracks. There was a man standing there with a gun pointed right at me.

Normally I am fairly brave, but now my blood ran cold. My mouth went dry. I knew I was an easy target for a man taking deadly aim at me. Hardly breathing I waited for him to fire. When he didn't, I called to him. There was no reply. So I moved toward him. Imagine my relief when I found that instead of a man with a gun, it was only a potted plant with a branch pointed towards me. It took a moment to get over the shock. When I could laugh, it was at being so frightened at what my imagination had done to me.

WE CHRISTIANS ARE LIKE THAT

We project our fears onto things we don't understand, then become afraid of them.

We can read about fasting in the Word of God; but because we've never done it, we imagine it to be something awful. We fear the unknown. Having no experience with fasting, it remains mysterious to us. So we impose our fears on it. When we do, it becomes the potted plant turned into a man with a gun. We imagine the worst, forgetting completely that God has given it to us.

Now I understand this fear. I've been over the fasting road a number of times and it is familiar to me. My fear of it is gone. But I remember how I felt the first time I tried it. I envisioned all sorts of terrible gnawing pains. I imagined hurting myself by going without food. This was in spite of the fact that everything I had read told me there was nothing to fear. It's just the idea of doing something for the first time. What I'm saying is this, I know how you feel.

You're wondering if it is something you should do? Will you be able to stand going without food? Does God want you to do it? Right?

● Let me share with you something that will be true for 99% of all who undertake a spiritual fast to gain control of their bodies. **There are FIVE PHASES a person goes through on an extended fast.** By extended I mean one of 20 or 30 or 40 days. You will NOT go through all these phases, but I want you to know about them. On a ten day fast, you will go through several of them. Did you know it is possible that you may feel so terrific at the end of ten days, you may wish to keep on going? That's right. And it will be OK if you do. But here's what you can expect:

82

THE FIVE PHASES OF FASTING

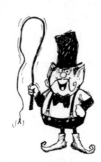

PHASE ONE . . .

HUNGER

For the first day or so, you will feel hunger. But it will NOT be because your body needs food. It can go for days and days without food, but that doesn't mean it will like it. Your stomach is used to receiving food regularly. It will kick up a fuss. It will act just like a SPOILED CHILD begging and nagging for what it wants. But you must ignore those cries. **They are the voice of HABIT**, the voice of APPETITE.

I'm not going to tell you it is pleasant or fun to go without food. But I think you'll be thrilled with the help the Lord gives. Also I think you'll be delighted to find out that it wasn't half as bad as you thought it was going to be. Lots of people testify afterwards, that it was a lot easier than they thought it was going to be. Some find a glass of water takes care of most of their hunger pangs. They only last for 15 minutes anyway.

Here's the hardest part—**WITHDRAWAL SYMP-TOMS.** That's right, when you fast you suffer these symptoms. Why? Satan has turned us into **"food-a-holics."** We're addicted to food. So when we quit eating, we go into withdrawal. Of course, the symptoms vary with each person. But usually everyone experiences something, even if it is nothing more than a headache. Others have feelings of weakness. Still more might feel a pain here or there. The point is, your body does react for a few days. But it won't be severe. Knowing it is a NORMAL part of fasting should take away the apprehension. The FEAR of **what might** lie ahead is the worst part. I'm hoping to remove that by describing the five phases.

PHASE TWO . . .

HUNGER LEAVES

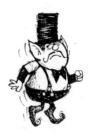

This may vary with the individual. The fact that all sense of hunger leaves in 48 hours is a natural phenomenon confirmed by medical men and fasting supervisors alike. It will bring you GREAT DELIGHT to discover this in your own experience. Why does it occur? The body can draw on STORED carbohydrate for about 48 hours. When that is gone, a chemical signal is sent from the pituitary gland into the blood stream. By a bit of chemical magic (known as ketosis) your body **shifts from burning FOOD as fuel and starts living off of stored fat.** The body begins to feed on itself—digesting its own fat! The body always needs fuel. Yet it is so designed that if it cannot get it from food, it will draw on reserves stored about the body. During the fast, YOU LIVE OFF YOUR OWN BLUBBER. There is no hunger because the body satisfies its hunger by burning its own fat as fuel. Food may still look good to you, but you'll have no craving for it. The craving is gone because the NEED is gone.

PHASE THREE . . .
WEAKNESS

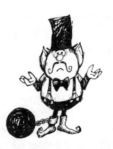

After the hunger leaves, you'll experience weakness for a day or so. For many this is the most difficult part. They don't like the weakness, for it seemingly takes a lot of effort for the simplest tasks. This could last as long as four days. Once it passes though, fasting is almost effortless. During the weakness interval, you may want to rest a lot. You should if you can. But you can be comforted by the fact that **during this time your body is throwing off the worst of its wastes and poisons.** When it's over, you're going to end up with much healthier organs. If the ten days end before your weakness is gone, don't worry about it. You'll still accomplish what we seek to do . . . gain control over the "spoiled brat."

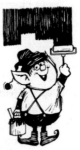

PHASE FOUR . . .
INCREASING STRENGTH

We come to the easiest part. The weakness is passing and your strength is returning. Fasting is routine from here on. You'll find you can return to your usual work. You have plenty of strength. You may have a bout of weakness now and then, but don't let that disturb you. Any such attack will pass shortly and fasting will seem almost effortless. You will have little or no concern for food. You feel as though you could go on fasting indefinitely.

In the Veterans Administration Center in Los Angeles, doctors have fasted obese patients up to 177 days, with little or no discomforts or serious side effects. In reducing programs at two Scottish hospitals, patients were fasted for 249 days with losses up to 97 pounds. Again no undue discomfort or distress. God has definitely designed the body to live off of its own stored resources for days with no ill effects. This is why it stores excess food in the first place. This is also why we get fat. The same God Who designed the camel to store water, designed us to store food. For the body to shift from burning FOOD to burning stored fat is as natural as can be.

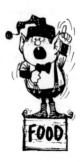

PHASE FIVE ...
HUNGER RETURNS

You won't do this, of course, but let's suppose you went on an extended fast of 30 or 40 days. How would you know when it was time to break the fast? No need for concern. The body has a way of letting you know. When the cleansing process is over and all the fats, wastes and bad cells have been eliminated, the body will then start feeding on HEALTHY TISSUE. When that starts to happen, **the body will sound an ALARM.** Why? Fasting has now ended and starvation is beginning to occur. The body SOUNDS A WARNING BELL. What is it? **THE RETURN OF**

HUNGER. That's right. When you come to the end of the fasting period, hunger returns and you know it's time to break the fast. That's why we noted the words in Matthew Four . . . "He then became hungry." Or as it reads in the KJV. . ."He was afterward an hungred" (Matt. 4:2). During the 40 days, the Lord experienced no hunger and was not tempted. Then came the warning signal—hunger. Now the devil had something to work with. And do notice that his first temptation had to do with FOOD.

● Since you are not likely to go on a 40 day fast, the WARNING SIGNAL will not mean much to you. But it is comforting, I think, to know that you can't go into starvation without an ALARM going off. Sometimes people will get this signal on the 21st day. It does vary according to the amount of fat stored in the system. In our program you'll be breaking the fast long before you get to that point. But I have explained it so that you'll have the whole story. Who knows, some day you may wish to go on an extended fast and get yourself a brand new body. Or should you ever find yourself trapped or isolated, it's precious to know you can go for days on nothing but water.

A quick review of the five phases of fasting:

PHASE ONE . . . HUNGER. You suffer the withdrawal symptoms of a "food-a-holic."

PHASE TWO . . . HUNGER LEAVES after the first 48 hours or so.

PHASE THREE . . . WEAKNESS up to four days. Body is throwing off worst wastes and poisons.

PHASE FOUR . . . INCREASING STRENGTH. The easiest part. You may find you can return to your normal work.

PHASE FIVE ... HUNGER RETURNS signaling end of fast.

ONE OF THE GREAT BARRIERS TO FASTING

There are hindrances to fasting. One of the greatest is NOT your hesitancy to try it, but the cautions and warnings of well meaning friends and doctors. They will not only try to KEEP YOU FROM FASTING, but invariably they will try to get you to break it, once you've started. They will tell you you're damaging your body or starving it to death. The devil will reinforce their words ... "You're going to hurt yourself."

It takes will power to resist them.

Doctors who oppose fasting (many do not) can come up with scary statements. Among the things they will tell you ...

There is mineral loss.

Protein loss, causing the hair to fall out.

Vitamins are excreted.

The body becomes highly acid.

The brain is deprived of sugar.

Metabolic machinery is overloaded with your own fat.

Low blood pressure.

Impaired kidney function.

Excessive loss of electrolytes in the urine.

Liver function threatened.

Headaches ... nausea ... and on and on.

Now there is SOME truth in all of these claims. Doctors aren't dumbbells. But there is something they refuse to face—God has built a fantastic intelligence into the human body. **The fast is GOD'S IDEA, not man's.** It certainly isn't the devil's. He hates fasting, knowing how it subdues the flesh. Since God designed the body for fasting, it is far wiser for the believer to take God's Word on it over the theories of doctors. Besides, the human body is always fooling our doctors.

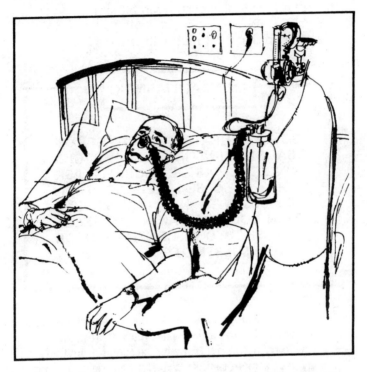

"He won't live another six months . . . !" How often have doctors said that, only to have their patients live YEARS longer. The body is SMARTER THAN THE DOCTORS. God made it that way. There is much our physicians still do not know about the body. They do not know how any hormone works, for example. They can only observe what happens. Fasting involves hormones. Now I'm not putting our doctors down. They're gifts from God and we're thankful for them. But they are just men. Remember the Karen Quinlan case? Her body was kept alive by life support systems. Her doctors said she would die without them. Her parents, wanting to let her die, went to court. The judge ordered the life support equipment disconnected. Did she die? To the embarrassment of the physicians, she remained alive for months after that. So our bodies are capable of far more than current medical expertise can fathom.

Having said that . . . I must still sound a . . .

MEDICAL WARNING

GO TO YOUR DOCTOR FOR A PHYS-ICAL EXAMINATION BEFORE BEGIN-NING THE FAST. BE SURE TO ASK FOR A GLUCOSE-TOLERANCE TEST. DISCUSS WITH HIM ANY MEDICA-TION YOU ARE TAKING TO SEE IF YOU SHOULD DISCONTINUE IT OR FIND A SUBSTITUTE.

NOTE. If you go to a doctor who is of a school opposed to fasting, he may try to talk you out of it. He may tell you to try it, but is sure it won't accomplish anything. He'll say that a more sensible way is to eat right. You already knew that before you went to see him. But eating right won't pull down Satan's stronghold or put you in command of your body. All you want from your doctor is the answer to one question: **"Is there any particular reason why I can't go on a 10 day fast?"** People with certain chronic liver and kidney diseases should not fast. Neither should those with diabetes or tuberculosis, or any with blood dis-ease or cerebral disease. Also it is not for pregnant women. For a normally healthy person, there shouldn't be any problem whatsoever. If you are anemic or hypoglycemic you definitely wouldn't want to try it on your own. But if your doctor is willing to work with you, he can keep you out of trouble. If he should say you have a disorder that makes it impossible to fast, either go along with him or find another doctor who knows the value of fasting and would be willing to supervise your fast.

● The safety record of fasting is remarkable. No other method comes close to it. Some authors claim there has never been a single death due to fasting. Yes, some have starved themselves to death, but that is not fasting. **Fasting** and **starvation** are two separate things. **Starvation feeds on good tissue, while fasting feeds on fat.** In rare instances people have died while fasting, but their deaths were **NOT caused by fasting.** Autopsies revealed the presence of organic disease as the cause of death. In terms of safety, fasting is without doubt one of the finest healing and corrective methods available to man.

So don't let fears instilled by friends and physicians rob you of one of the greatest experiences God has for you. Our bodies, with their organs and appetites, are wonderful servants. But as Derek Prince says, "They are terrible masters." They have to be brought under subjection and KEPT THERE. Every Christian undertaking a fast for the purpose of bringing his body into subjection, is saying to that SPOILED BRAT . . . "You are the servant, I am the master."

SUMMARY

Fasting is the most powerful attack we can launch against the FOOD JERICHO Satan has built in our minds. There's no way to allow such a stronghold to stand and hope to gain control over your weight or eating habits. A person will be plagued the rest of his life if he by-passes this fortress. This is why diets won't do. Our assault on JERICHO has to be with **no food at all.** This is the quickest and most effective way to bring the body into submission.

The fear of fasting fades when you learn that hunger disappears after 48 hours of no food. There will be withdrawal symptoms, because we are food addicts. The most bothersome, perhaps, is weakness that you feel while the body is detoxifying itself. Once weakness passes, fasting is pleasant. There is no danger of starvation.

The body has its own ALARM SYSTEM—the return of hunger. Usually this alarm doesn't sound until 20 to 40 days of fasting, depending on how fat a person is. Ten days is well within safe limits. Once you get your medical clearance you're ready to go. So let's get started. That's next.

CHAPTER SIX

Going On The Fast

"I humbled my soul with fasting. . ."
(Psa. 35:13 NASV)

THE FIRST DAY—GETTING STARTED

It's Monday morning, the day you have chosen to begin your fast. The weekend is behind you. It has been a sane weekend. Knowing the fast was coming up, you tapered off on self-indulgence. You backed away from coffee and tea. This is not because it is necessary to condition your body for a fast, it isn't. But it is good to prepare yourself psychologically. The most important preparation is that of your mental and emotional attitudes. A person can go abruptly into a fast without any prior emptying of the system or attempts to sweeten it. What really helps is **coming to the fast without fear.** Beyond that if you are looking forward to some FUN WITH THE LORD, it can be a great experience. A little self-denial can heighten your anticipation.

As you prepare to rise in the morning, the first thing you do is sit on the edge of the bed. You greet your heavenly Father:

"Well Father, today is the day we start taking control of this body. I thank You for showing me that it is up to me to do this. However, since I can't do anything without You, I ask You to lead me and help me. You are the expert, so I put myself in Your hands."

NOTE. Naturally you don't have to use those words. They're here simply to give you a feel for starting the day with Him. You are probably not even awake yet, so there's no need to be pious or profound when you speak to Him. He expects you to yawn. The idea is to start the day with Him. Here's a powerful hint: when your "spoiled brat" starts acting up, demanding food, use those impulses or desires as SIGNALS TO PRAY. You don't have to stop what you're doing. Just chat with the Lord as you go about your business. There will be times when you might say, "Lord, it's a little rough right now. How about a boost to get me over the hump?" You may say that often during the first 48 hours of the hunger interval.

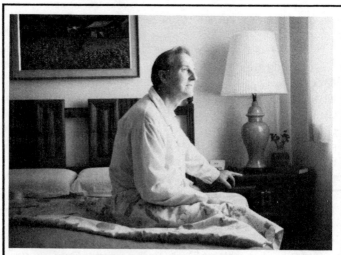

As you prepare to rise in the morning, the first thing you do is sit on the edge of the bed and greet your heavenly Father.

• As you make your way to the kitchen, head for the sink. A glass of water will do for breakfast. It's surprising how satisfying water can be. And isn't it nice to have breakfast out of the way so fast? No dishes either, except when you may have to clean up after your family.

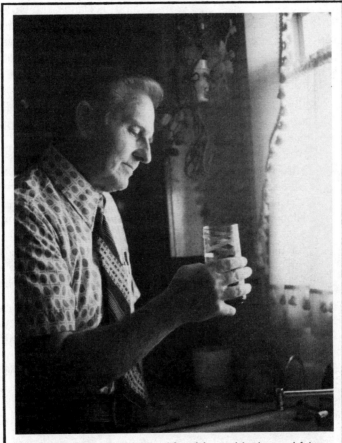

A glass of water will do for breakfast. It's surprising how satisfying water can be.

The first time I went on this kind of a fast, I didn't experience hunger until late that afternoon. Water carried me along nicely. When my wife and daughter sat down to the table, I went off to my room. Their conversation and those good smells were getting to me. The "BRAT," (my appetite) began making his customary demands and I got some real insight as to how spoiled he was. I thought to myself . . . "Man, am I hungry!" Then it struck me . . . "Wait a minute! Hasn't the Holy Spirit revealed to you that your body can go without food for weeks?" I wasn't all that hungry. It was Satan putting the pressure on my appetite. And he didn't stop there. I could hear his whispered suggestions . . .

"Why don't you forget this nonsense, CS, and go in there and eat with your family. You keep this up and they'll think you've gone off the deep end."

HINT. You can take the sting out of that suggestion. How? By anticipating your family will have such feelings. Before you begin your fast, announce your intentions. Do it far enough in advance for them to have time to understand your motive. Since you are doing this "as unto the Lord," for the purpose of bringing your body under control, they can't fault your motive. If the members of your family are Christians, they'll admire you for it. They might even be encouraged to follow your example.

My first time out, the devil was really busy with his temptations. Once he got me to think about eating, he did everything he could to arouse the EATING IMPULSE within me. Every time he'd come with one of his suggestions, I'd deal with him and the impulse would subside:

"Satan, in the name of Jesus, take your suggestions and get out of here. I want God's blessings, not your temptations. So I command you in His name to depart from me, for it is written . . . "Delight thyself in the Lord and He will give thee the desires of thine heart!"

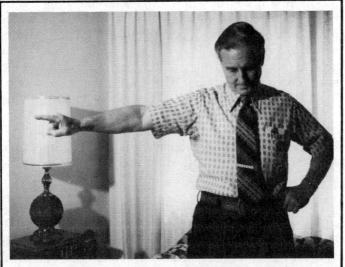

"Satan, in the name of Jesus, take your suggestions and get out of here. I command you in His name to depart from me!"

● It's amazing how much authority we have over Satan. And it's FUN to use. When you start something like this for the Lord's sake, you have plenty of spiritual backing. The devil knows we're on the road to power and self-control and he works furiously to hinder us. That's why this book began with instructions for dealing with him. Want to know what happened when I ordered him away like that? He left immediately. The evidence was a marked release in the pressure on my appetite. This happened every time I commanded him to go. I knew God was going to see me through the fast.

What About Side Effects?

Since we're going through the first day, this is a good time to mention the bothersome side effects of fasting. There are some. They're unpleasant. But they're tolerable. I experienced some of them, but they weren't too uncomfortable.

97

The first is bad breath. Within a few days the tongue becomes coated and your breath is offensive. This is true of all who fast. The lungs throw off lots of poisons which are discharged into the air as you exhale. To be able to mix socially, carry a little bottle of breath-sweetener. There are a number of them on the market, but I use Listerine's mint flavor. You merely touch the tiny bottle to the tip of your tongue. The solution is strong enough to last for quite awhile. Some are made with a nozzle and can be sprayed into the mouth. Either type will keep you from offending and will help to make conversation more pleasant.

Other possible nuisances (besides weakness which we will discuss more fully on the fourth day) are **dizziness, fever, headaches, nausea, cramps, weak-knees, shortness of breath, sleeplessness, backache, runny nose, and pains in various parts of the body.** I know all that sounds terrible, but you will only have one or two of them. The only reason I state the whole list is that in case something shows up as a result of your fasting, you won't be alarmed by it. If you didn't know in advance, you might think you were damaging your body in some way. Satan will try to make sure that's exactly what you think.

So relax. It will be normal. The symptoms will pass as the condition causing them clears up. Actually, **some of these symptoms are brought on by the HEALING PROCESS taking place in your body.** One thing you might watch for is getting out of a chair too fast. You're more prone to dizziness so don't jump up too quickly.

> **NOTE.** During a fast your body temperature usually remains constant. But it is easier to feel a chill. Always keep your body warm. You may find you want a blanket over you on a summer night. It's also a good idea to do a few little exercises before you get out of bed. This moves the blood a bit and will help prevent dizziness as you rise. If you get up too fast, your head could spin. Another common complaint is headaches. Those who give up coffee and tea

for the fast (and they should) sometimes experience withdrawal symptoms. This is because the caffeine present in both is a drug. You can get a head start on these symptoms by going without tea and coffee a few days before you begin the fast. Some people like to get over their withdrawal headache before they start fasting.

THE SECOND DAY

On the **second day** my hunger pangs were worse. Each time I had a real attack (which only lasts about 15 minutes), I'd go to the sink and get a glass of water. Then I'd say to the spoiled brat . . . "There, that'll hold you." Amazingly the body would settle down. Then I'd order Satan away. It is thrilling the way the Lord backs our commands to the devil. The stress subsides quickly and everything becomes quite manageable.

NOTE. The second day and night may be the most difficult. As the available carbohydrate is used up and the body has to shift to stored reserves, you approach the worst of the hunger attacks. This varies in each of us. Some people feel they just have to eat something, others find water quite sufficient. If you are one who feels the second day (the crisis hunger) will be too rough for you, then you will appreciate SIDE TWO of the **FASTING CASSETTE**. On this cassette, you and I take a glass of water, go find a comfortable place where we can stretch out and chat about the wonderful things happening to you as you fast. It is called . . . "GETTING OVER THE HUMP" (No. 544). That's exactly what it does. Together we work through the hunger attacks. At the same time I demonstrate exactly how to deal with Satan when he tries to tempt you to eat. You don't need this cassette to use the plan in this book . . . but if you want extra help until your hunger leaves, the cassette will give it.

The second day was the most difficult for me. Yet, it wasn't as bad as I thought it would be. My fears proved groundless. The glasses of water, persistent dealing with the devil and little chats with the Lord got me through

99

the day and night just fine. Things do go better with Christ. When the hunger passed, I felt I had fought . . . AND WON! From that point on, I knew it was going to be down hill all the way. For someone else, though, the weakness of the fourth day may prove to be the hardest part.

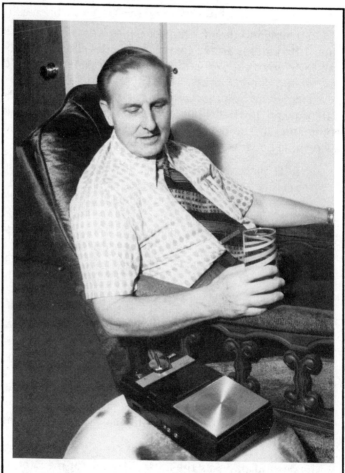

Here's a fantastic way to get over the hunger hump—a cassette and a glass of water—really powerful help.

DON'T CHEAT. You will ask, "Aren't there times when I'll be tempted to sneak a nibble of something? Surely a bite or two of some fruit couldn't hurt anything, could it?" There will be times when you're tempted to sneak a snack, but you just can't give in to the temptation. Why? Your body is in the process of shutting down the entire digestive system to live off of STORED NUTRITION. You're not going to be living off of food for awhile. Your body is gearing up to burn fats and wastes as fuel. So if you eat ANYTHING THAT HAS TO BE DIGESTED, no matter how small the amount, it will cause gastric juices to flow and the digestive system will have to be cranked up again to handle it. To eat **ANY food, after the 48 hours,** is like driving along and suddenly throwing your car into reverse. It will foul up the whole process. So plan on taking nothing but water.

THE THIRD DAY

By the **third day** there was a marked decrease in my hunger. The cries of the flesh subsided considerably. The SPOILED BRAT had settled down. The worst was over. To be honest with you, the idea of hunger bothered me more than anything else. Why? I have a huge appetite and little will power when it comes to food. I'll bet there are lots of Christians just like me . . . some who won't even go on diets because they're afraid of being hungry. So I was very relieved when the hunger passed. The side effects, which might bother others, didn't trouble me half as much as the fear of being hungry. I guess that comes from being part of a society of gluttons.

THE FOURTH DAY

With the passing of hunger, you know your body is starting to live off of fat. As it shifts to this different kind of fuel, there will be a few days of weakness. Knowing about this weakness in advance really helps. It takes the mystery out of it. You may even find yourself saying . . . "Well, Lord, things are going just as we expected, aren't they?" In the midst of any weakness, ask the Lord to strengthen you for any tasks which **just have to be done.** If you work at a job demanding hard labor, you should take off for a few days until your strength returns. Right at this point your body is going into a **cleansing crisis.** Very heavy amounts of toxins and wastes are being incinerated and the "ashes" eliminated. You are running on pretty low grade fuel.

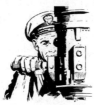

FUEL. Familiar with submarines? When a sub runs on the surface of the water, it is powered by diesel engines. These engines deliver lots of power which propel the submarine along at a good rate. It can do so as long as the fuel lasts. When the sub dives to run submerged, it operates off of batteries. Battery power is **stored** energy. It is limited. It can't take the sub very far or very fast. When the battery power is gone, the sub has to surface and run off the diesel engines. Fasting is something like that. Normally, we eat 3 times a day and have more than enough good fuel. We even store the surplus. But when we fast, we're like the submarine running on its batteries. We're then operating off of stored energy. It is LOW GRADE FUEL. It consists of fats and wastes and poisons converted into energy. It's not the greatest energy source for running a body, but it is adequate. Because stored fuel is LOW GRADE we don't get the same performance out of it as we do when FOOD is converted to energy. This accounts for the weakness a person feels, also for those times when he might feel chilly. It is nothing to worry about. The Lord has designed us to run off of this fuel as surely as a sub is designed to run off of her batteries.

What About Working, Then?

There's no reason why a person shouldn't go to work, if he feels he has the strength to do his job. He is going to function at reduced capacity because of the LOWER grade fuel. But if his job is not too demanding, he should be able to do it. However, during the two or three days when the body is consuming the WORST of its wastes and poisons, there is a good chance he won't feel like doing anything.

The weakness felt during the "cleansing crisis," depends a great deal on a person's physical condition, his age, and state of mind. Of those three, I feel his state of mind is the most important. The man or woman going into the fast, trusting the Lord for MINIMUM DISTRESS, will pass through the weakness period with far less discomfort than the person approaching it fearfully, expecting the worst. Very often, what we EXPECT to happen, has a lot to do with what does happen. That's why I'm giving you such detailed information. Take advantage of it. Use it to develop a positive attitude toward fasting. There is no danger. Besides, it can be fun to watch yourself go through the different stages of the fast.

What About Body Wastes?

As you may know, the body disposes of its wastes in four different ways:

❶ THROUGH THE SKIN. Did you know that our skin is the largest organ of the body? A lot of wastes pass through its millions of pores. This is greatly increased during a fast. Therefore frequent bathing is needed to wash away the wastes and to keep the pores open.

❷ THROUGH THE KIDNEYS. The kidneys have the task of cleansing the blood stream. With so much waste material being thrown off at this time, one might think extra water would be needed to keep the kidneys flushed. The best opinion is that natural thirst is a good guide. Usually the desire for water is not great during a fast, but if you take 5 or 6 glasses a day, that would not be excessive. It varies with the individual, ranging from one pint to two quarts. If you have access to well water or bottled spring water, that is best. Distilled water can be used too. Try to avoid chlorinated tap water.

❸ THROUGH THE LUNGS. We've already mentioned the bad breath due to the toxins and wastes discharged as you exhale. This will be particularly true during the weakness period. The blood stream brings considerable poison to the lungs to be discharged into the air. As much waste material passes through the lungs as through the kidneys, bowels and skin.

OFFENDING. Some people head for the woods when they fast. If they are experienced fasters they know the peculiar odor given off by the lungs is offensive. However, the breath sweeteners available today are so efficient it really isn't necessary to hide out any more. A tiny drop on the tip of the tongue, mixed with a lot of saliva, will cover the odor for some time. It is so diluted in the mouth, that it won't trigger any gastric excitement when it finally reaches the stomach. But chewing gum is another matter. That is taboo. There is almost enough sugar in an ordinary stick of gum to interrupt the fast.

❹ THROUGH THE BOWELS. You may think your bowels have gone on strike. They shut down very quickly. Your last movement should occur about 24 hours after your last meal. Then the system takes a nap. You could possibly have one more movement, but once the contents are discharged from your digestive system, that's it. Don't worry about it. Your bowel system will enjoy the rest. And it will be rejuvenated by the cleansing process.

ENEMAS. Some books on fasting recommend enemas. But most physicians are against them. They say that fecal matter left in the bowel will do no harm, even if it stays there for weeks. They don't like the idea of flushing away the protective mucus that lines the walls of the colon. However if a person has eaten some refined foods that do not easily pass through the 25 foot long bowel, he could have some dried out material that could generate gas and make him uncomfortable. I favor an enema when anything in the bowel distresses you. It will relieve you psychologically and that is important. If a fasting Christian believes he could harm himself through impaction of some material that would be hard to pass when the fast is over (or simply makes him feel plugged up), he will be apprehensive. He won't enjoy the fast as he should. An uneasy mind is a hindrance the devil can use. However, if you are comfortable, forget about enemas. Your body knows what it is doing.

FIFTH AND SIXTH DAYS

Let's say you have experienced weakness for three days. That would take us through the **fifth day.** On the **sixth day** you feel strength returning. Ah, but it won't be the same strength you had before the fast. Remember, you're running on a lower grade of fuel. Don't expect to be able to go full blast for the remainder of your fast. You still have to baby yourself. Figure on functioning at ¾ of your usual capacity. Your body will appreciate it.

WEIGHT LOSS. What's happening to your bathroom scale now? Something you'll like. If you play the game honestly (taking no food at all) you will lose about 2 pounds a day for a week. It may happen for the whole ten days. It all depends on how much fat you're carrying. It is possible to lose TWENTY POUNDS in the ten days. But keep in mind this is merely a BY-PRODUCT of our fast. **Our primary purpose is the destruction of the FOOD STRONGHOLD Satan has built in your mind.** It's going to come down, too. The cry for food has ceased. There may be times when the fragrance of food will give you a queasy stomach. You can expect the condition of NO HUNGER to remain stable until the stored reserves are exhausted or you decide to break the fast and awaken the digestive system.

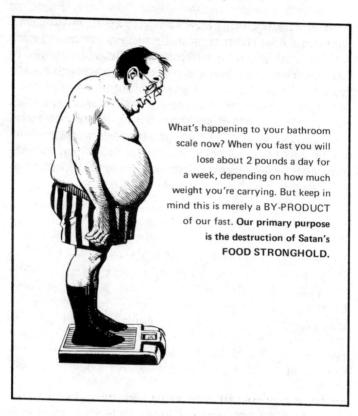

What's happening to your bathroom scale now? When you fast you will lose about 2 pounds a day for a week, depending on how much weight you're carrying. But keep in mind this is merely a BY-PRODUCT of our fast. **Our primary purpose is the destruction of Satan's FOOD STRONGHOLD.**

THE SEVENTH DAY

You'd think the fast would be routine by now. **But with the silencing of your flesh, your spiritual appetite is on the rise.** A fascinating shift occurs in your prayer life. The Lord seems so much closer to you. It's as though you could reach out and touch Him. You lose track of time as you talk to Him. You achieve an intimacy never possible when your flesh was actively pressing its demands. You get the feeling you could ask and receive almost anything from God. You thrill to a new power in prayer.

● It can be fun to watch yourself pass from the carnal state to the spiritual state while fasting. I'm dwelling on this so that you'll be looking for it. It is fascinating to see your flesh die down and your spiritual appetite zoom to a height you've never known before. From that point on, fasting becomes an exercise in communion. Well, it should be. I would be disappointed if Christians used this book merely to lose weight and didn't care to draw closer to the Lord. Our ability to rise above circumstances is in direct proportion to our closeness to Christ.

Think of all the times your family will be eating and you will be off by yourself. Spend that time with Jesus. Because of your heightened sensitivity, you'll notice things about Him that escaped you before. You'll feel His passion for you. His presence can become almost overpowering. You'll love Him so much, you could just "eat Him up." Fasting can bring you into a glorious intimacy with the Lord that cannot be attained any other way. So don't think to yourself, "Now what am I supposed to do while the rest of them are eating?" Look on it as prime time to draw close to Jesus and do things in prayer you could never do otherwise. It is the greatest force available to man. What then must it be like for the person whose spiritual sensitivity has been quickened! It's too wonderful to waste.

HAZARD. Due to the subsiding of your flesh and your heightened spiritual awareness, you become sensitive to the spiritual realm. But you're not only sensitive to the Holy Spirit. You also become vulnerable to satanic suggestion. The devil is aware of your increased sensitivity. So be suspicious of any dream or vision (these often come during fastings) **that tends to EXALT SELF in any way.** Open to the entire spirit realm, you will be able to receive **BOTH satanic and divine impressions.** Any vision that is truly from

God will exalt Christ, not you. Any word of prophecy you receive must be checked against God's Word. The devil would like to send you off on a tangent. If you thought you had received something special from God, when it was actually from Satan, you could be deceived. The devil is a great counterfeiter. So don't make any changes in your life work or relationships with others or embrace different doctrines BASED ON VISIONS ALONE. Check everything against the Word before making such decisions.

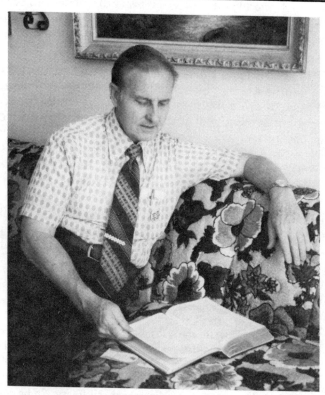

Think of all the times your family will be eating and you will be off by yourself. Spend that time with Jesus. Fasting can bring you into a glorious intimacy with the Lord that cannot be attained any other way.

AS WE COME TO THE END

The **8th to the 10th days** find you stronger physically. You can do chores with comparative ease. Hunger is no problem. You may wish to go beyond the 10 days. If your doctor says it is OK, and you really want to, by all means do so. You'll see some amazing things take place in your body if you do. However, most of you will be anxious to return to eating. There are too many things going on around you in which food plays an important part. Relatives come to visit, there are parties and outings, events at church involving food and even trips are planned. Eating plays such a part in life's routines that 10 days is about all the average person can manage. For some, even that is a great sacrifice.

● Your days of fasting will pass quickly if you appreciate your increased spiritual sensitivity and spend more time with the Lord. I hope you enjoy HIM so much, you'll be reluctant to awaken your fleshly appetites. It can be exciting to work with the Lord when He seems close enough to touch. And that's how it is when the flesh is out of the way. But of course, you have to return to eating. When you do, the closeness of the Lord will diminish as your drives and passions come to life again. What we hope is, as we come to the final phase of this plan, that your commitment to Christ will be such that you'll be able to retain much of the control you've gained through the fast. To the degree that you are successful in doing this, to that same degree you will enjoy a closer walk with the Lord.

> **CAUTION.** From earliest times it has been recognized that fasting was God's way of conquering the body and mastering the appetite. This is why David says, "I afflicted myself with fasting" (Psa. 35:13). Believers fast for many reasons: to get answers to prayer, deliverance from demons, physical healing, seeking the mind of the Lord, etc. But the reason you're fasting is to gain control of your body that you might present it to the Lord. It is something you're doing

FOR HIM as well as for yourself. Therefore, **to keep your motive pure, do not make an outward show of your fasting. Keep it to yourself and your family.** Otherwise Satan might tempt you into an outward show of piety, as if to say . . . "See how spiritual I am. I'm on a fast." If Satan can get us to use the fast to glorify ourselves, he will have demonstrated his control over us in a most sacred area. The wisest policy is not to say anything, lest our words indicate a desire "to be seen of men" (Matt. 6:5). For the man who really wants the victor's crown, fasting is the swiftest way to go.

When it is time to break your fast, **some caution is needed. How you come off of a fast is more critical than how you begin.** It has to be done gradually. Why? Because of the colon and stomach. Both have been shut down for 10 days and need to be **eased** back into action. If, for example, you broke your fast with a large potato, it might pass solidly into the intestinal tract. From there it might have to be removed by surgery. You wouldn't want to go through anything like that. Your organs are NOT READY for solid food. They need to be started up again and it has to be done carefully. We look at that, next.

FINAL NOTE: This plan is based on a 10 day fast. But if you feel it's impossible for you to go without food for that length of time—don't get discouraged. The Lord has an answer for you. If you'll turn to the two very back pages of this book, you'll find "ADDED HELP." I'm very excited about the breakthrough we've had in fasting and the discovery of the fasting powder that makes it possible for many to fast, who couldn't otherwise do so. Also you'll find there a suggestion for creeping up on fasting by doing it in steps. That way you don't have to plunge for 10 days your first time around.

CHAPTER SEVEN

Breaking The Fast

"I have broken my spirit with fasting. . ."
(Psa. 69:10 NEB)

Did you know that animals fast? A female bear, for example, takes no food at all during her hibernation. She may even give birth to a cub and have plenty of milk for it, long before she starts eating again. Where does this come from? Not from outside sources, surely; but from a store of nutritive materials inside her body which adequately serves her for months.

When a dog is ill, he will go off some place and hide. He will lie down in a dark, quiet place and go without food. You could put a plate of food in front of him but he won't touch it. Guided by instinct, he goes on a fast. He wants to be left alone while his body cleanses and repairs itself. He might take a sip of water now and then, but that's all. When his fast is over, he carefully nibbles at any food that might be handy. But as you watch him, you see he is in no hurry to get a lot of food into his stomach. Only gradually does he return to regular eating.

Where do animals get this wisdom? The Lord created them with the knowledge already built into their computers. No animal thinks to himself, "I'm going on a fast to get well." Neither does he realize how careful he has to be when he comes off the fast. He is simply doing what his body tells him. The point: God programs animals for fasting, and He also programs them for breaking the fast. When we watch them break their fast, we see how gingerly they return to normal eating.

● Had the Lord designed us so that our eating and fasting habits were regulated by instinct, I wouldn't be writing this chapter. We'd automatically do what our bodies tell us. But we're not creatures of instinct. That is, our bodies are not supposed to tell us what to do. It is the other way around. God wants us in charge of our bodies. He has designed us after His image, as creatures who THINK. That way we decide what is best, not our bodies. This means it is up to us to USE OUR HEADS when it comes to eating and fasting. When we think about it, what is more obvious than the fact that care is needed in breaking a fast.

WHY CARE IS NEEDED

When we stop eating, our bodies make dramatic adjustments. Three things happen:

(1) the stomach shrinks far below its normal size and the gastric juices cease to flow;

(2) the organs involved in digesting food (intestines) go into hibernation;

(3) a whole new energy process is activated as the body converts from a food-burning machine to a fat-burning machine.

Now those are significant changes.

If a person went on a long fast, say 30 days in dura-

112

tion, he'd get a new stomach out of the deal. His rejuvenated stomach would be just like that of a baby's. Even
on a 10 day fast, those organs enjoy a deep rest. Care is
needed in bringing the digestive system out of hibernation and getting it back into full operation. Common
sense tells us that.

> **NOTE.** With the stomach arousing from its nap it will not
> be ready to handle solid food. It will take almost 3 days be-
> fore things are back to normal. If a person tries to break his
> fast with solid food, the digestive system could rebel. The
> stomach may not digest it at all. It will then be passed along
> to the small intestine which isn't ready for it either. There
> it could remain to generate gas and bring on a lot of distress.
> However, since we are coming off of a TEN DAY fast, there
> is always the chance the system might accept it, but only
> because it was shocked into action. Even then it will be far
> from its power of normal function. Your organs will appre-
> ciate it if you give them a few days of special care rather
> than abuse them. They will reward you with problem free
> digestion if you show them this courtesy.

● **Nearly every authority in the field of fasting agrees
the safest way to break the fast is with juices—either
fruit or vegetable.** Not only are juices easily digested but
they are easy on the linings of the stomach and intestines. These linings become very sensitive during the
fast and are almost certain to react to anything abrasive.
The best way is to start with **uncooked** juices. Most supervisors prefer unstrained orange juice as the one that
seems to get the bowel action started most easily.

If you do not have access to **fresh** orange juice, then
apple juice will do, or tomato juice or grape juice. **BUT
DON'T USE MILK.** It's harder to digest and not easily
processed in the lower intestine if you get too much at
once. Some people have a little trouble with milk after a
fast. So give yourself a few days before you take any.
The fruit and vegetable juices stimulate the gastric juices
in the stomach and gently wake up your lower digestive

tract. One of the best vegetable juices is carrot juice.

HINT. A day or so before it is time to break your fast, start laying in the juices and items you'll be using to awaken your digestive system. If you don't have a juicer, try to borrow one so that you can have freshly extracted juices. There are vitamin substances that last only minutes after squeezing and with a juicer you can avail yourself of them. If melons are in season, you'll want some of them too. If you have to get carrot juice at a health food store, do so. It's only for a few days. **Try not to use cooked, canned or bottled juices.** The fast can be broken anytime, day or night. It may be needless to say the body now needs truly wholesome food, though not too much of it. You can understand that **junk foods are out.**

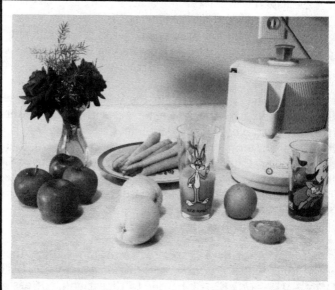

Nearly every authority in the field of fasting agrees the safest way to break the fast is with juices—either fruit or vegetable. The best way is to start with **uncooked** juices. If you don't have a juicer, try to borrow one so that you can have freshly extracted juices. Try NOT to use **cooked, canned or bottled** juices.

YOUR FIRST FOOD

FIRST DAY

Pour out ONE-QUARTER glass of fruit or vegetable juice. Add an equal amount of water to make it half-strength. It should not be cold, but room temperature. THEN BEGIN TO **SIP IT**. Don't gulp it down. If you downed four ounces of fruit or vegetable juice at this point, it could induce cramps.

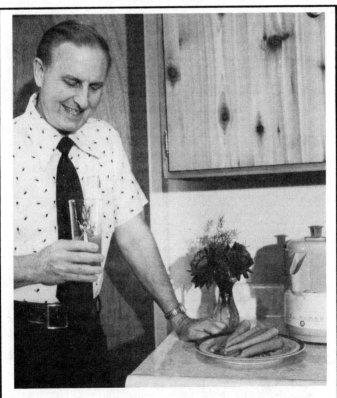

On the **first day** of breaking your fast, pour out ONE-QUARTER glass of fruit or vegetable juice. Add an equal amount of water to make it half-strength. Then begin to **sip** it.

An hour later, sip another HALF GLASS. You shouldn't experience any discomfort at all. An hour later take a FULL glass. If you feel any discomfort, go back to the half-glass for the rest of the day. If there is no discomfort, then try a HALF-GLASS of undiluted juice. Should that bring discomfort, go back to the diluted juice for the rest of the day. Do not take more than one pint at any one time.

SECOND DAY

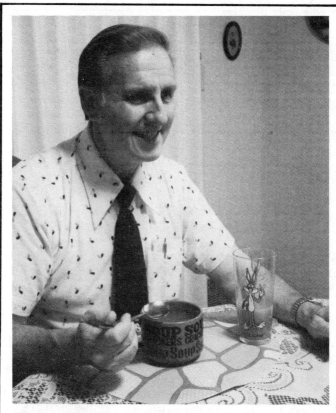

On the **second day** try some soup for lunch. It should be clear soup not made with milk. Also avoid any broths made with meat.

Take one pint of juice for breakfast. Again, sip slowly. Try to "CHEW" the juice. Sounds funny, but this allows the acid and sugar of the juices to mix with the saliva to make it a lot easier on your stomach. It won't have to work hard to handle it, being eased back into action gently.

For lunch try some soup. It should be clear soup not made with milk. Also avoid any broths made with meat. Strain the soup to take any solids out of the stomach. There is no hurry. Take small amounts. If any bloating occurs, go back to juices again.

For dinner try a little fresh fruit. It could be an orange or a grapefruit. If melons are in season, a small amount of melon would be good: the equivalent of an orange. If fresh tomatoes are in season, you could eat one. But it must be well chewed.

THIRD DAY

Breakfast can include any of the fresh fruits in season. But don't overindulge. The stomach won't want to handle very much. Don't let Satan tempt you into overdoing it . . . "Man, I'm going to make up for lost time." That's what he wants you to think. But don't push your tummy. If you feel you are overworking it, back off. Go to juices again for the remainder of your meal. Try a baked apple.

Lunch can now include a very small fresh vegetable salad. It won't need any dressing, unless you want to put some lemon juice on it. A cooked, non-starchy vegetable (leafy greens) could be added. Doesn't sound like much of a meal, but your stomach doesn't want too much right now. Try a little cottage cheese with your salad.

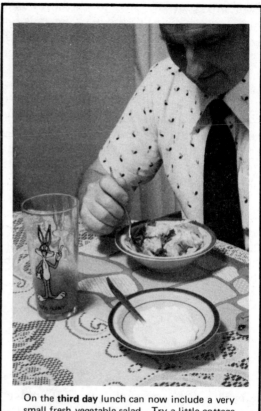

On the **third day** lunch can now include a very small fresh vegetable salad. Try a little cottage cheese with it.

For dinner a light meal of fruit. The amount can be a little bigger than what you had for breakfast. A plate of selected fruits can be very filling at this stage.

FOURTH DAY

Fruit again for breakfast. Lunch can now include a salad and a baked potato. Or make that a baked apple, if you prefer. Protein may now be introduced in the form of cheese or eggs, if you find your body is accepting the food well.

Fresh fruits are eaten again for dinner, but toasted whole grain bread may now be eaten with a thin scraping of butter. You can add some milk now, preferably raw, nonfat milk. If you experience any discomfort from the milk, return to juices, skipping the next meal if you don't feel like eating. You have to play it by ear at this stage.

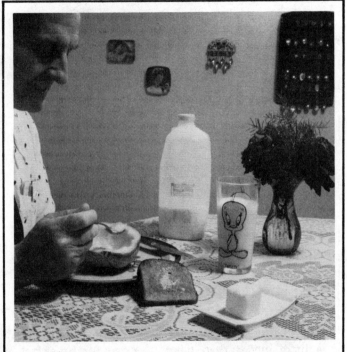

On the **fourth day** fresh fruits are eaten again for dinner, but toasted whole grain bread may now be eaten with a thin scraping of butter. You can add some milk now, preferably raw, nonfat milk.

FIFTH DAY

By now you should be returned to normal eating. The caution now is HOW MUCH you eat . . . and

HOW you eat it. Your food should be chewed to the point where it is practically liquid before it goes into your stomach. **At the first feeling of fulness—STOP.** Remember, we want to EDUCATE your body to live on far less food than it has been used to in the past. It is good to say to yourself . . . "Big meals are out for me."

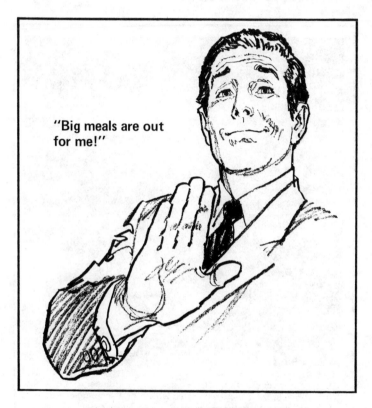

"Big meals are out for me!"

NOTE. Weight returns quickly after a fast. You're going to be shocked when you see HOW LITTLE food is needed to keep your weight at the level you reached through fasting. If you plan to keep on going down, there is no way you can return to your former eating habits. When a person stops eating, large amounts of water are eliminated from the body. This accounts for much of the loss. The bathroom scale isn't aware of the reasons. A pound is a pound as far as the scale is concerned. It doesn't distinguish between fat, water or wastes. You're going to like what you see in the mirror. You look different, you feel different. Regardless of what makes up the weight loss, you feel better and look better.

Picture your digestive system as cleansed and rested. It is now ready to extract the most out of everything you eat. With that in mind, you won't be surprised to discover you can hold your weight on as few as 600 calories a day. Now that is a very low amount. I don't suggest that you try to live on that amount. But eating lightly is part of the process or re-educating your body concerning food. You're in command now. You're the boss. Your body is to get what it **needs,** rather than what it **wants.** You're through catering to that "spoiled brat." To maintain your control, determine to keep your eating down to a minimum . . . somewhere around 1250 calories a day. Most readers will still have pounds to lose.

AFTER FIVE DAYS

Your system is working again and you can handle most foods once more. But do you want to put **poisons** back into a body you've just cleansed? Of course not. Some foods on the market today are **pure poison.** Since you are going to be living on reduced fare for a time, you don't want those 1250 calories to be made up of bad foods. When your intake is restricted, it is more important than ever that the foods you do eat supply your body with the nutrients it needs.

This is NOT a book on nutrition. But I must mention the bad foods and explain what makes them bad. They contain lots of calories yet are devoid of the elements needed to keep your body healthy. Some are truly poison, loading your body with toxins to the place where your health is endangered. Since there are so many good foods you can eat, I should first of all list those you should avoid.

FOODS TO AVOID

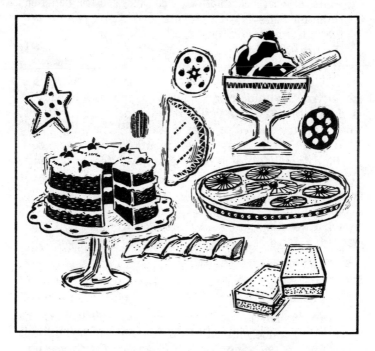

Refined sugar products: jams, jellies, ice cream, jello, cake, candy, chewing gum and soft drinks (except diet drinks).

White flour, bleached flour, enriched flour: white bread, biscuits, buns, cookies, pastries, gravy, noodles, pancakes, waffles, spaghetti and pizza.

Catsup and mayonnaise.

Salt: salted foods, potato chips, crackers and french fries.

White rice and pearled barley.

Fried foods.

All foods cooked in or containing saturated fats and hydrogenated oils.

Coffee, decaffeinated coffee, tea, alcoholic beverages, chocolate and cola drinks.

Smoked foods: lunch meats, hot dogs, salami, bologna, pastrami and bacon.

Packaged breakfast foods. (Shredded wheat is acceptable, grape-nuts second.)

> **NOTE.** We're going to be talking more about the things you should not eat. Chapter Eleven will zero in on them to the place where you may get serious about eliminating them from your pantry. But I'd like to sow a seed in your thinking. When the various magazines coming to your home feature articles on nutrition, read them. It's time for you to bone up on nutrition. There's quite a bit to learn. Some good books are appearing on the market as the result of studies conducted by universities. While the medical profession will be slow to change, (it is a good thing doctors don't jump at everything that comes along) various publishers are making a lot of good material available to the public. You'll be smart if you plan on becoming your own nutritionist. I am planting that idea in your mind now, hoping it will grow as we proceed through the rest of the book.

SATAN'S HOLD IS BROKEN

Let's consider what you've accomplished with your fast so far:

❶ **Satan's hold on you through food has been broken. For the moment you are in the driver's seat. The challenge now is to KEEP IT.**

❷ **You've tasted what it is like to have your fleshly appetites subside, allowing you to draw closer to the Lord. You find yourself more eager to do His will** than anytime since you were first saved.

❸ You've lost some weight, feeling better probably than you have for a long time. You see a different image in the mirror. You are satisfied it is within your power (with the Lord's help) to be trim and attractive.

• Don't spend too much time congratulating yourself. Satan is watching. He has a sly smile on his face . . . "Let the sucker gloat. He'll get careless and I'll have him fat again before he knows it." You see, he believes he can make you fat and keep you fat. Your temporary victory doesn't worry him. He's seen many ride the yo-yo. They lose a lot of weight and then put it all back on again. He thinks he's got it made. So you're not surprised when I tell you it is important to **WATCH OUT FOR HIS ATTACKS ONCE YOU START EATING AGAIN.**

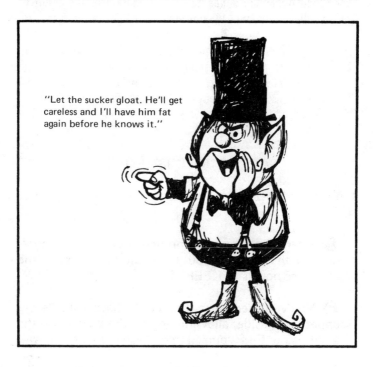

"Let the sucker gloat. He'll get careless and I'll have him fat again before he knows it."

Your first food will cause your body to shift back to a FOOD-BURNING machine. As long as you are living off of stored energy (burning up fat) there is no hunger. But once you awaken the digestive system, **the hunger signal returns.** The devil knows that. What he doesn't know is that you are coming off this fast with the idea of **LOSING MORE WEIGHT.** You're not going back to your former eating habits. **You're still on the program.** The fast has merely put you in command of your body.

There has yet to be devised a program that will keep weight off the Christian who resumes his bad eating habits and allows his appetite to dictate what he eats. So if you have any thought of using the fast to lose weight and then feel you have it made, you might as well quit right now. You're doomed to failure. The uniqueness of this approach is that we use the fast **MERELY TO BREAK SATAN'S HOLD.** Then we continue on a program calculated to keep us in command of the body.

Plan on losing MORE weight after the fast is over. We want you lean and trim. At the same time, we are going to **CHANGE your attitude toward food.** You're going to learn to eat differently . . . and be programmed to do it the rest of your life. Why the rest of your life? Because the food problem never goes away. We will be eating until we die and if there is plenty of food around, the threat of getting fat is ever present. The only hope for keeping you slender and trim is **PROGRAMMING you with new eating habits.**

● In the back of the book is an **"ENERGY EQUIVALENT CHART"** showing in MINUTES how long it takes to burn up different amounts of food. You may wish to remove the pages to hang on your kitchen bulletin board. If you get some of these values fixed in your mind, it can take some of the fire out of Satan's suggestions. It's easy to put fattening stuff in your mouth, but so hard to get it off of your body. Here is one way to blunt the edge of Satan's attacks. A good look at this chart should convince you WHY your eating habits must change.

NOTE. If you don't already have a kitchen bulletin board, you'd better buy or make one. There are going to be several items you'll want posted for quick reference. A glance at the energy chart shows what a slight indulgence can lead to. A large banana, for example, contains about 100 calories. Depending on the program you adopt for yourself, you may only be able to afford one a week. If Satan can get you to EAT TWO OF THEM, the 100 extra calories have to go somewhere in your body. If you indulge in an extra 100 calories a day on desserts (a low figure really) you'll gain 3500 calories or one pound in a month's time. Keep that up for a year and you'll be 12 pounds overweight with a single habit. Remember your body is a calorie counter. If you indulge in something during that same 24 hour period, you'll have to GIVE UP something else of equal caloric value . . . or you'll get fat.

WHERE ARE WE GOING?

DOWN. And to continue going down after you come off the fast, you're going to have to become aware of the caloric content of the various foods and your absolute LIMIT on calories needed to maintain your weight. I know that sounds like a big job, but you'll be surprised how quickly this comes to you. In time it will be second nature for you to know which foods you can and cannot afford to eat.

We're headed to the same weight you had when you were 22 years old. Assuming, of course, you were lean at that age. If not, then you'll be going down to the weight shown on the standard weight table for your height, age and frame. To do this requires a knowledge of what food is all about and what it can do. That information is going to be part of your new life-style. AND . . . you're going to be programmed to live accord-

126

ingly. That'll mean more to you when we come to **PHASE III** of the plan.

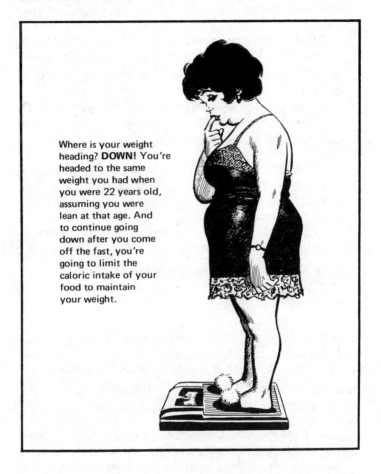

Where is your weight heading? **DOWN!** You're headed to the same weight you had when you were 22 years old, assuming you were lean at that age. And to continue going down after you come off the fast, you're going to limit the caloric intake of your food to maintain your weight.

● When I speak of your newly programmed life-style, here's the kind of information that is going to regulate your life:

▪ **You will know and eat nutritional foods of low caloric value.** Most people think that food is food, totally unaware that much of what they eat has NO FOOD VALUE at all. Just because they feel full, they think they're feeding their bodies. They're not, of course, because there's so little nutrition in what they eat. So living on nutritional foods **only** will be a new concept.

■ **You will gear yourself to moderate eating** . . . taking smaller portions . . . eating slowly . . . disciplining yourself to leave a BIT OF EVERYTHING on your plate. It is a powerful technique to say "I QUIT" the instant you feel comfortable. To continue eating once hunger has been appeased is to be a slave of appetite.

■ **Avoid liquids that are high in calories.** If you must have coffee, learn to drink it black. Sugar and cream add too many calories.

■ **Agree with the Lord that you are going to eat only those things which make for a healthy and slender body.** And that you're going to do so just to please Him.

■ **Take note of the proper weight for your age.** Experiment to determine the number of calories that will hold you at that weight. STICK to that amount. Of course you'll be eating less than that until we get you to your proper weight level.

■ **Explore new taste sensations.** Develop a liking for foods with a low fat-making potential. Make a game of it and do it with the Lord. As you try a new food say, "Lord, what do you have for me in this?"

■ Are you the family cook? Do you sample foods for seasoning? Don't let Satan deceive you into thinking those samples should not be counted as part of your meal. Those few calories add up faster than you think and Satan knows it. And he specializes in TINY AMOUNTS. A wee imbalance in calories can trigger

128

a dangerous habit that will eventually make you over-weight.

ALARM. If for some reason you should find yourself TWO POUNDS overweight, allow your spirit to become ALARM-ED. Call on the Lord and take ACTION IMMEDIATELY. The quickest way to deal with the emergency is to MISS MEALS. Your body will object, naturally. But you've learned by now that your body can miss a lot of meals with no ill effect. Besides, you're in command now. Your body has nothing to say about it. The pleasure of eating a meal or two is not to be compared with the far greater satisfaction of looking nice for the Lord. So be prepared to MISS MEALS when the scale says Satan is about to do it to you again. A TWO POUND increase over your proper weight level should turn off all eating for a meal or two. Believe me, that is the BEST WAY to keep yourself at the right weight level when you see that scale starting to creep up on you.

SUMMARY

You've won a great victory with your fast. And now you're coming off of it. Winning one battle does not mean you have won the war. Historians point to the Battle of Dunkirk when Hitler had the British army broken and trapped on the beaches. He failed to press his advantage and eventually lost a war he had virtually won.

You have snapped Satan's hold on you by your 10 day fast. You now have him on the beaches of Dunkirk. If you relax your vigil and permit him to regain lost ground, you could lose the war. That would put you right back where we started . . . and you'd have to go through it all again. So be prepared to WATCH the food frontier. **Condition yourself to THINK THIN . . . EAT THIN . . . FEEL THIN . . . ACT THIN.** I'll be showing you how to do that.

We have now covered TWO PARTS of the plan: **(1) we've**

learned how to detect and deflect Satan's food darts; (2) we've broken his hold with the fast. We have yet to PROGRAM you to eat to live rather than live to eat. The program has to go into your MIND, since the mind controls the body.

We go into the control room . . . NEXT!

PHASE THREE

How to re-program yourself for proper eating habits

You have now come to the most important part of this book. All that you have read to this point has been preparatory. There is no way to achieve permanent weight control, without programming yourself for proper eating habits. In the next four chapters you'll be learning how to do this programming.

CHAPTER EIGHT

Welcome To The Computer Room

"For as he thinks within himself, so he is."
(Prov. 23:7 NASV)

 Were you to visit our facility here in Baldwin Park, one of the places you'd pause on the tour would be our computer room. You'd see blinking lights, hear the sound of whirling discs and a printer would start up all by itself. As you watched, that printer would pour out endless names and addresses on a long folded sheet. Millions of names are in that computer—yours no doubt among them.

As you stepped inside the doorway, your tour guide would say . . . "This is our computer room."

The guide would point out the various pieces of equipment about the computer room, but he wouldn't have to tell you a lot about them. They are so much a part of life now, nearly everyone is familiar with them and what they do. They perform quickly and without emotion. Yet all computers are bound by a rigid law—they can respond only to what is put into them. **Computers cannot think for themselves:** they can only react.

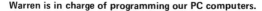

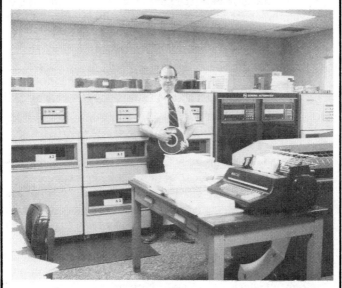

All computers are bound by a rigid law: they can respond only to what is put into them. Computers cannot think for themselves—they can only react. Therefore they have to be PROGRAMMED to tell them what to do.

The technique for putting information into a computer and telling it what to do with that information is known as PROGRAMMING. We've used that word a number of times already.

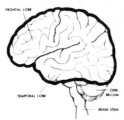

Did you know that the human brain is a fantastic bio-computer? That 3 pound organ which God has placed inside our heads is actually an amazing piece of machinery. Believe it or not, the Lord has written some astounding programs for this computer and they are all in operation when we're born into the world. This is why so many of our body functions are fully AUTOMATIC.

NOTE. The **brain** is the controller, organizer and information processer of the body. It is the **BOSS.** Even though it makes up but 2% of the body's weight, it gets 20% of its blood supply. It gets its share of the nutrients in the blood stream before any other part of the body. No matter what is going on anywhere else, the brain is supplied first of all. **This is why we don't have to worry about starving the brain on a fast.** It looks out for itself. The brain has complete control of many of the life processes of the body. This is why we don't tell our hearts to beat or how fast. The brain automatically keeps the body at 98.6 degrees fahrenheit and has the complete oversight of our digestion, elimination and circulation. It even sends signals directing the kinds of acids and enzymes going into the stomach as well as the proteins our bodies manufacture. While it may seem that you and I are in charge of our bodies, literally thousands of functions are regulated by this computer . . . right down to the blinking of our eyes. Nearly every process is computer-controlled, most of which we are totally unaware.

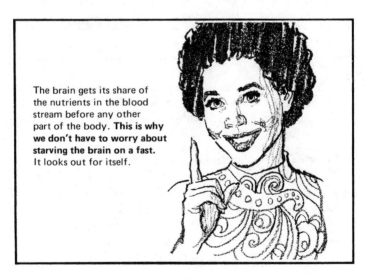

The brain gets its share of the nutrients in the blood stream before any other part of the body. **This is why we don't have to worry about starving the brain on a fast.** It looks out for itself.

● Man has two levels of mental experience—**conscious and unconscious.** In the conscious he does all of his thinking, planning and deciding. At the conscious level he is aware of himself and his surroundings. He has no idea of what is going on in the unconscious (subconscious), for it functions by itself. The Lord has designed man so that certain aspects of his being operate wholly beyond his awareness. Things go on in a person's spirit, for example, which he can sense, but he can't put his finger on anything. It is all BEYOND his awareness.

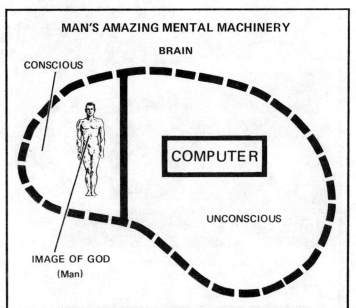

MAN'S AMAZING MENTAL MACHINERY

BRAIN

CONSCIOUS

COMPUTER

UNCONSCIOUS

IMAGE OF GOD
(Man)

See the two compartments of the brain? The conscious is shown with the figure of the man standing. While the conscious mind is used for thinking, planning and deciding, **the UNCONSCIOUS is the computer.** There is no way for a man to invade the computer room so as to see what is going on there. The Lord has sealed it off from awareness. It is because it is beyond awareness that it is called the unconscious. While the conscious shuts down when a person sleeps, the unconscious (subconscious) never shuts down. The regulation of the body requires constant care. All of the functions mentioned above, i.e., temperature, circulation, and digestion of food must be maintained by the computer round the clock.

THE COMPUTER—GOD'S SUBSTATION

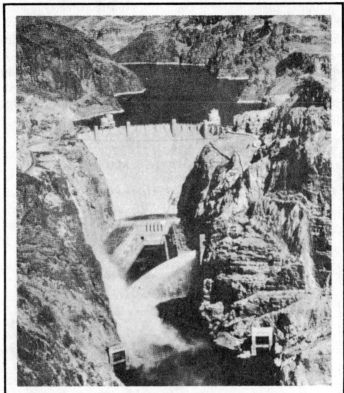

Aerial vew of Hoover Dam and Lake Mead at Boulder Canyon of the Colorado River where it forms the boundary between Arizona and Nevada.

Come with me to Hoover dam. As we tour the different levels, we come to the mighty generators that produce electricity for Southern California. This is the PRIMARY source of power for our area. That power travels across the desert in huge cables strung on giant steel towers. When it arrives in the Los Angeles area, it is divided among various substations from whence it flows to industry and individual homes.

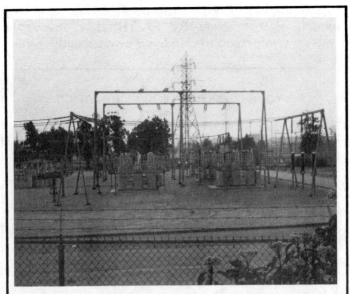

When power arrives in Los Angeles from Hoover Dam, it is divided among various SUBSTATIONS. From there it flows to industry and individual homes.

God's power flows something like that. The agency by which power from God comes into our lives is the Holy Spirit. He dwells in every believer (Rom. 8:9). **He ministers that power THROUGH OUR COMPUTERS** making them something like SUBSTATIONS. This means that every Christian has immediate access to the power of God. Keep in mind the computer works at the spirit or unconscious level. If a person wishes to avail himself of the power of God, he must plug into his own computer—by faith.

Stated another way, **it is by means of the COMPUTER that God makes His power available to His people.** This means our unconscious computer is MORE THAN A MACHINE. It is linked to God through the Holy Spirit. Since the computer is also spirit, **it is connected directly to the SOURCE.** If a believer wants to do something in the power of God, he can do so, but he must avail himself of that power—**BY FAITH.** If he doesn't, he ends up trying to do the job in his own strength.

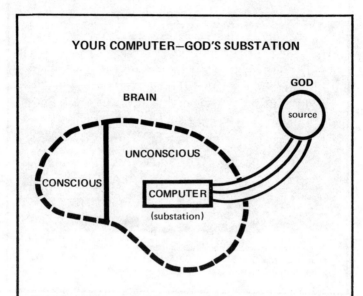

YOUR COMPUTER—GOD'S SUBSTATION

Power comes from God into our lives through the Holy Spirit who dwells in every believer. **He ministers that power THROUGH OUR COMPUTERS,** making them something like SUBSTATIONS. Don't let all this talk of CONSCIOUS and UNCONSCIOUS bother you. You needn't remember any of it. The only reason it is mentioned is to let you know that God's power is available to help you control your eating habits as well as maintain the health of your body. If you remember that much, you can forget the mechanics of how it works. If you can picture your mind as a substation for the power of God, you'll have the essential truth.

 Remember the old wash boards? You'd stand it in the tub and rub the wet clothes on it. That's the way my grandmother used to wash clothes. But today we plug a washing machine into the electrical outlet and our clothes are washed for us by a power-operated machine. There's a big difference between washing clothes by hand and doing them in a machine. Similarly there's a big difference between trying to over-

138

come weaknesses and habits in our own strength, rather than in God's power. One way is fairly easy, the other almost impossible.

● Why do I say that? I want you to start thinking of **your computer as GOD'S SUBSTATION.** Later I'm going to suggest a WHOPPING CHANGE in your eating habits. When you face the kinds of foods that must go out of your life, your first thought will be . . . "No way. I couldn't possibly do that!" But when you consider that God has a power substation built right into our computer, what might otherwise seem impossible is actually easy. Letting your computer take over and do something for you in God's power is a lot different than trying to do it in your own strength. Believe it or not, WE CAN USE the computer—by faith.

WE CAN PUT PROGRAMS INTO THE COMPUTER

While the Lord created us with specific programs written into our computers for the automatic regulation of our bodies, **that doesn't prevent other programs from being added afterwards.** Indeed all kinds of programs can be entered into the computer. We add them ourselves from time to time. Usually we do so without realizing it, because it is done INDIRECTLY. Inasmuch as we are BARRED from the computer room, we cannot do any DIRECT PROGRAMMING. With the computer beyond our awareness, we have NO DIRECT CONTACT with it at all. But we are able to insert programs **indirectly** and sometimes they have a serious effect on our bodies. The LAW which covers this phenomenon reads like this:

WHAT WE CONSCIOUSLY BELIEVE TO BE TRUE, OUR UNCONSCIOUS MIND (THE COMPUTER) ACCEPTS AS FACT. AND WHAT IT ACCEPTS AS FACT, IT SEEKS TO CARRY OUT IN OUR BODIES.

In other words, if we believe something to be true with our conscious minds, the subconscious portion of the brain accepts it as fact and tries to execute it in our bodies. This means:

OUR BODIES EXPERIENCE REACTIONS ACCORDING TO WHAT WE BELIEVE, RATHER THAN TO THINGS AS THEY REALLY ARE.

Here's a roomful of women chatting gaily over tea. Someone screams . . . "A mouse . . . !" The whole group turns into a mob of shrieking, scrambling females trying to escape. Understand, there doesn't have to be a mouse. All that is necessary is BELIEVING a mouse is present and you have panic. If the ladies believe a mouse is there, the FEAR RESPONSE is automatic. Suggestion alone is enough to trigger the reaction. Why? The ladies are PROGRAMMED to react this way, probably from years before. Now if all those present THOUGHT IT WAS A JOKE, that there really was no mouse, everyone would have remained calm. It was what the ladies BELIEVED that produced the panic.

See—our bodies react to what we **believe.** That's a LAW.

THE LAW OF BELIEF

A student, thinking to play a prank on his teacher, hides a rubber snake in her desk. You know what will happen. The snake isn't real, of course. But when the teacher opens the drawer, the rubbery thing quivers, looking very much alive. Her eyes spot the wiggling reptile and her mind screams . . . "SNAKE!" No judgment is made as to whether or not it is real. She believes one thing . . . "It's a snake!" Instantly PRE-PROGRAMMING takes over. The fear of reptiles is already in her computer. So what will she do? Shriek and leap back from the IMAGINED DANGER.

Does it matter that the snake is made of rubber? No. It is **WHAT SHE BELIEVES** that counts . . . not the real truth. It doesn't matter a bit that it is just a harmless toy. Her body doesn't respond to the facts, only to what she believes. She believed the snake to be REAL and that's all that was necessary to make her computer go into action. The computer you see, responds according to the **LAW OF BELIEF.** Here's the law again: **what we consciously believe, the computer accepts as fact.**

● A lot of things happened in that teacher's body because of what she believed. The computer caused her pulse to quicken. Adrenalin poured into her bloodstream. Her stomach closed off. All digestion ceased abruptly. Muscles tensed throughout her body. Her entire being was geared for danger . . . **and it was all AUTOMATIC.**

> **BIBLICAL NOTE.** God delights in showering His blessings on all men. But He has ordained that those blessings should come to people by way of established laws. Not all of His laws are mentioned in the Bible. Some, like the laws of electricity, gravity and aerodynamics have to be discovered. When they are, they can be used. Then they become God's blessing to all who use them. Other laws, such as the law of the harvest (sowing and reaping) are found in the Bible. Since the LAW OF BELIEF has to do with human behavior we would expect it to be in the Bible also. And indeed it is. It is expressed in numerous ways, but a precise statement is found in Proverbs 23:7 . . . **"As a man thinks in his heart, so is he."** That is, what the mind believes ("thinks in his heart") is ultimately expressed in his behavior ("so is he"). Finding this LAW in the Word of God gives us the confidence to use it.

 A friend of mine is forever saying . . . "Everything I eat goes to fat." He really believes that. Considering what you have just learned about the LAW OF BELIEF, what do you think my friend looks like? You're right. He's as fat as he can be. He's using the law of belief **negatively.** He believes the food he eats is making him fat, so his computer accepts that belief as a command and seeks to carry it out in his body. There are people who honestly BELIEVE FAT-NESS is a way of life for them. As long as they continue to think that way—AND BELIEVE IT—the law guarantees they will STAY FAT. Until they get a **different image** of themselves, their computers will do their best to turn every bit of food they eat into fat. And nothing will change that. It's a LAW.

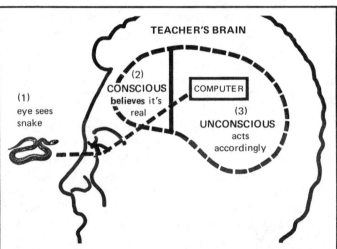

TEACHER'S BRAIN

(1) eye sees snake

(2) **CONSCIOUS** **believes** it's real

COMPUTER

(3) **UNCONSCIOUS** acts accordingly

Did the teacher tell her body to gear up for emergency? No. She DIDN'T give one command to her body. Everything that happened occurred **automatically.** All she had to do was **believe** the snake was real. From then on, the amazing computer in her unconscious took over. It caused her body to behave as it did. None of it was voluntary. But see this: the computer ordered these changes in her body **BECAUSE OF WHAT SHE BELIEVED!** As far as her computer was concerned, that snake WAS REAL. The computer has no eyes. It depends solely on the conscious mind for its information. If the conscious mind BELIEVES a live snake is there, the computer has to respond to that idea. Therefore: what we consciously believe, our computers **UNCONSCIOUSLY** seek to express in our bodies. This is a POWERFUL LAW, one we're going to use in controlling your weight.

142

THE TV SCREEN IN OUR BRAIN

Did you notice I said they need a **DIFFERENT IM-AGE** of themselves. But where will they behold this image? On the **SCREEN of the imagination.** We see lots of things on that screen. In fact, this is where we do all of our thinking and dreaming. When we see something on this SCREEN OF THE MIND and believe it, that's how we influence our body's computer.

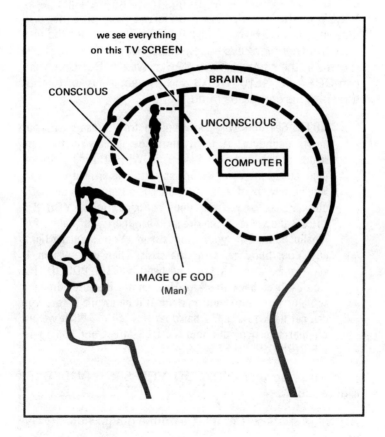

Here are the steps:

1. We consciously put a picture on the screen of our

imaginations.

2. We BELIEVE what we see there.

3. The computer accepts that SCENE as being real and responds accordingly.

• Here is something truly fascinating. **Man is able to do what no other creature can do—IMAGINE.** Made in the image of God, he can **CREATE** things on the screen of his mind. He can see things that DO NOT AS YET EXIST in the world. Man is different from all other animals in that he **THINKS** ON A SCREEN. All sighted animals whether monkeys, dogs, birds, bees or flies . . . have screens in their heads. They **SEE** as we do. But only man can **CREATE NEW IDEAS** and project them onto that screen in his conscious mind.

> **NOTE.** See now why we wake up from dreams with our hearts pounding? A terrifying scene appears on the conscious screen and you believe it. Why? During a dream, your conscious defenses are at rest. The critical and challenging powers of your mind subside during sleep. So, without any challenge from your conscious mind, **YOU BE-LIEVE** the scene in the dream. Fear stabs your being. Adrenalin pours into your bloodstream. Your stomach tightens. Your body gears for the crisis. Then you awaken. It was just a dream. Ah, but your heart is STILL POUNDING. You can't go back to sleep. How come? Because adrenalin **actually went into your system.** It'll be awhile before you can get back to sleep. What does this tell us? What we put on that screen of our minds DOES affect our bodies—IF WE BELIEVE WHAT WE SEE!*

• **Knowing that—HOW DO YOU SEE YOURSELF?** I'm serious.

"Oh, I suppose I'm a little on the plump side." (May-

---

*We've just touched on the highlights of our computer in this chapter. For those interested in a fuller treatment, please refer to the author's book **JESUS WANTS YOU WELL.**

be you chuckle a bit) "But I feel good. I guess I'm a few pounds overweight, but it's not all that bad."

That's what you say to me. But what do you REALLY THINK? How about when you stand in front of the mirror with no clothes on? Do you like what you see? Are you pleased with that? Be honest. Deep in your heart aren't you saying . . . "That doesn't look good. I'm too fat. I should do something about it?"

It's what you REALLY think about yourself that counts. If you **BELIEVE YOU ARE A FAT PERSON,** your computer will organize your body's resources to **MAINTAIN THAT IMAGE.** That's the negative side of the law of belief, or at least it is using the law of belief negatively. If you SEE yourself as fat—and believe it— that law says you will **STAY FAT.** God's laws, you see, are rigid, inflexible. They work in a very calculating manner. If we use them positively, they bless us. If we use them negatively, they punish us. It is important to keep in mind they work both ways.

If you forget everything you've read so far in this chapter, it won't matter. I simply wanted to expose you to the fact that what we BELIEVE affects our bodies—and explain why. You do NOT have to master this information to use the plan.

NOW FOR THE IMPORTANT PART
OF THIS CHAPTER

If believing the wrong image of yourself can keep you fat, what would happen if you stopped thinking of yourself that way and began seeing yourself as **SLIM**

AND TRIM? Then if you could bring yourself to **BELIEVE IT**, your computer would accept it as a command and your body forces would be geared to **MAKING YOU THIN.** Isn't that an exciting idea? Imagine having a powerful tool right there in your own brain that you can use to take off excess weight and keep it off. That's the great blessing God offers in this book.

This is not a "hope so" or "maybe so" matter. We are working with a fixed law and the power of God. God's laws do their work regardless. So you don't have to puzzle about this, or even be wishful. I can almost hear you saying,

> "How wonderful it would be if everything is as Brother Lovett says. It would thrill me no end to learn that God has a LAW we can use to regulate our weight; and His power is available to overcome our bad eating habits."

You can relax, dear reader. When you work with God's laws, you can't miss. You might as well accept it as fact—your weight is going to go down and stay down. We're not talking about a reducing diet or a fad diet. We're talking about a LAW God has established within us, one He wants us to use. Here's what that law means to you:

IF YOU CAN VISUALIZE YOURSELF AS THIN— AND BELIEVE THE IMAGE YOU SEE ON THE SCREEN OF YOUR MIND—THE LAW SAYS YOU WILL BE THIN.

Isn't that fabulous? You bet it is. It's time we started thinking about your new image and how to believe it. That's next.

SUMMARY

You've got a fabulous computer in your head. This amazing

146

piece of mental machinery regulates and controls every function in the life-process of your body. It is also a **SUBSTATION for the power of God.** Since a believer is joined to God through the Spirit, God's power is MINISTERED through the computer. This makes the power of God available to the Christian for overcoming weaknesses and habits as well as doing mighty works in His name.

Located in the Christian's UNCONSCIOUS, the computer is beyond his awareness. Thus he can't see it, or touch it. Neither can he make direct contact with it. But he can insert programs into it once he learns the Law of Belief. Now if that seems a little technical for you, all you have to do is keep in mind the snake story or the mouse story. They demonstrate the LAW OF BELIEF and that is all you really need to know. Here it is again:

WHAT WE CONSCIOUSLY BELIEVE, OUR COMPUTERS UNCONSCIOUSLY SEEK TO CARRY OUT IN OUR BODIES.

Remember—the actual condition doesn't matter. It is what you BELIEVE that sends the computer into action. The snake wasn't real, neither was the mouse. But that had no effect on the computer. It responds only to what a person believes. Its only contact with what is taking place is that TV screen; the one on which you see everything. When you **BELIEVE** what is on that screen, the computer does too . . . and goes into action. That's all it has to work with. It has no contact with the physical world.

Here's what this means to you. If you can develop a **NEW IMAGE** of yourself, one that pictures you as **trim and attractive,** it won't matter one bit that you are 15-30-50 pounds overweight. The truth is you could be 100 or 300 pounds overweight and it would make no difference. Your computer operates entirely by faith. Thus you can have rolls of fat hanging on your body and still visualize yourself as slender and firm—and if you BELIEVE THAT IMAGE, your computer will go to work to reproduce that new image in your body.

Now that is a terrific bit of information. Later on I'm going to be asking you to do things which **you think** can't be done, especially when it comes to giving up certain kinds of foods. But you can IN THE POWER OF GOD available through your computer. You will be able to program yourself for eating habits that will keep your body trim and attractive . . . and the computer will do the hard part for you. That may sound farfetched right now, but take my word for it . . . faith can go where reason cannot follow. A lot that God has for us must be appropriated by faith.

Now to learn how to do it.

CHAPTER NINE

Dare To Believe It

*"I tell you, then, whatever you ask for in
prayer, believe that you have received
it and it will be yours."*
(Mark 11:24 NEB)

Years ago, men infected with Malaria would shake with cold and burn with fever. Apart from wiping their brows and keeping them covered, little could be done for them. In some instances men suffered beneath the very trees that could heal them. Unknown to them, those trees contained the very properties that would ease their distress and bring the disease under control.

Then one day a poor Indian crept down to a spring where one of these trees had been overthrown by the wind and fallen into the water. The Indian drank the water. It was bitter, but his thirst made him drink it. Lo and behold it cured him of his Malaria. Some of his friends drank the water and they too recovered. Thus **quinine** was discovered. God had the remedy available all along, but without the knowledge of it, men sickened and died. There was a cure in the bitterness of those trees, but it had to be discovered.

• It has ever been so with the laws of God. It is the pleasure of our heavenly Father to conceal a thing that we might have the joy of finding it. The **LAW OF BELIEF,** central to PHASE THREE of this book, has been around as long as man himself. But only in recent times has man laid hold of it and sought to make use of it. Norman Vincent Peale, for example, is one who has exploited this law with his "power of positive thinking." But we're applying it to the holy task of looking trim and attractive for the glory of the Lord.

 Recently I received this note from a lady:

"Dr. Lovett, I have been overweight for 30 years. I desperately need to lose 80 pounds. My weight is giving me serious health problems, such as angina, high blood pressure and arthritis in my feet. I've had nine operations because of my overweight condition. I read your article, *THE DEVIL WANTS US FAT,* and I'd give anything to believe God has help for me. I am the most miserable Christian you've ever met. I would be eternally grateful to the Lord if you could help me."

Can you feel her agony? I did. So I took time to encourage her through the mail. I laid out for her a program, similar to the one in this book. It was abbreviated, of course. The thing that encouraged her most was the fact that she could work with the Lord. She had tried so many fad diets and weight loss clubs that she lost all hope of finding anything that would do the job. Because she was a Christian, her hope returned when she realized this approach was of God.

I said to her:

"If you can visualize yourself as TRIM and BELIEVE IT—your body's computer system will cooperate in bringing it to pass. Believing is the hard part, but when

you know something is of God, you have every reason
to be confident."

CONFIDENCE IN GOD'S LAWS

A man kills a young girl. Arrested and brought before the judge, he protests, "I didn't kill the girl. My hands did!" At once you suspect he is mentally disturbed. And you'd be correct. No man in his right mind so divides between his body and mind that he thinks his hands carry out acts independently of his thoughts. Only the psychotic thinks that way.

Can we divorce God from His laws? Can we say a LAW does this or that independently of God? Whether it is a law of nature or a law of human behavior, it can not be anything but God working out His purposes. All of God's laws are an expression of His nature in some way. That's what makes them reliable. The **LAW OF BELIEF** issues from God's nature as surely as any other law.

This is why a Christian can come to this program with confidence. It is solidly based in law. If you meet the conditions of the law, it will do its job. That is the nature of laws. They do their work implacably, irresistably. Therefore when I ask people to **SEE THEMSELVES** as slim and slender . . . **AND BELIEVE WHAT THEY SEE** . . . this law will work for them. It cannot fail.

● In view of what we have seen so far, you have ample basis for using the law of belief. Everything we have considered is **lawful** and **biblical**:

❶ God says "Resist the devil and he will flee from you" (Ja. 4:7). With what I have given you, **you can recognize Satan's food attacks and order him away.**

151

Thus a big eating pressure is removed by carrying out a biblical injunction.

❷ Through fasting you have gained power over your own body. In fact, pounds have come off as a result of taking authority over the "spoiled brat." This too is in accordance with God's Word . . . "I buffet my body and make it my slave . . . " (I Cor. 9:27). Again, you're working with solid biblical law.

❸ You've learned that your computer CAN be programmed for a NEW IMAGE; one that sees you slim and trim. Inasmuch as . . . "ALL THINGS are possible to him that believeth," I am challenging you to put a new image on the screen of your mind and DARE TO BELIEVE what you see (Mk. 9:23). God's law says if you believe it, it will come to pass (Mk. 11:23, 24).

● As you VISUALIZE yourself as TRIM AND AT-TRACTIVE a **NEW IMAGE** is fed into your computer. If you truly believe what you project onto the screen, your computer will **ACCEPT IT AS A COMMAND.** Then the forces of your body will be geared to making that trim image a reality. From this moment on, determine to do just that. And do it with confidence, knowing you are making use of a divine law.

NOW LET'S GET STARTED

Here are the two stages: (1) **putting the image on the screen,** that's the easier part; (2) **and believing what you see on the screen.** That's the harder part. But that is what it is going to take. So how shall we start?

ACTION

With no clothes on, stand in front of your mirror. You don't like what you see. I know that. But we've got to start some place. If you have privacy when you get up in the morning, do it then. If you have to wait until bedtime, that's OK too. Here's what I want you to try. You're going to look at your body with the EYE OF FAITH and **reshape** that image so that you see yourself as you'd like to be . . . a **perfect specimen.** Sounds impossible? You wonder how you can change your body simply by looking at it. It's something you do with the Lord. So close your eyes for a moment . . .

"**Lord Jesus, help me use the Law of Belief for your glory!**"

● You know what we're attempting, don't you? All right. Eyes still closed, try to picture yourself as trim and attractive. I mean, see it on the screen of your mind. Slowly open your eyes and look in the mirror again. Can you see any changes as you look at your body? Any changes at all? None. Okay, close your eyes again and go back to the image on the screen of your mind. Take a good look. Now open your eyes once more and look in the mirror. Any changes now? Still none? That's all right. Go back and forth like that for a while.

After you've gone back and forth 8 or 9 times you'll begin to project your new image onto the mirror . . . **with the eye of faith.** You'll see **some** changes. Work with this MIRROR EXERCISE until you get some change. Do some later in the day, if possible. Again at night. And tomorrow and the next day. In time you'll be able to look in the mirror BY FAITH and behold the same attractive image that appears on the screen of your imagination.

This mirror exercise is our starting point for working with the computer. Since faith can go where reason cannot follow, we are able to see things with the eye of faith as **THEY ARE GOING TO BE,** rather than **AS THEY ARE** at the moment. God does this, you know. He sees things before they come into existence. Since we're His image, we can do the same . . . but **BY FAITH,** of

153

course. That's the difference. With this exercise, we work both your faith and your imagination. It is an experiment in PROJECTING what you see in your mind's eye. And along with it, developing the faith to believe what you see. This exercise flexes your faith and your imagination.

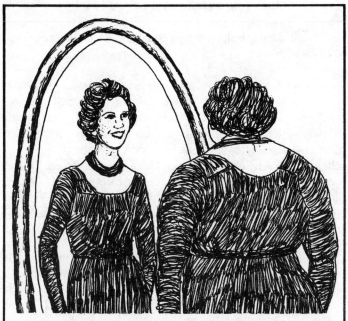

Soon you'll begin to project your new image onto the mirror **with the eye of faith.** This mirror exercise is our starting point for working with the computer—**by faith.**

During the Day

From time to time throughout the day, close your eyes and practice putting the NEW IMAGE on the screen of your imagination. A dozen times for the first few days wouldn't be too many. You'll get good at it in time. Keep in mind we are making use of a God-given tool. Few people take their imagination seriously, let alone make purposeful use of it. What a waste. Well, you're not going to waste yours any longer. You're going to make good use of it, even if it seems awkward at first.

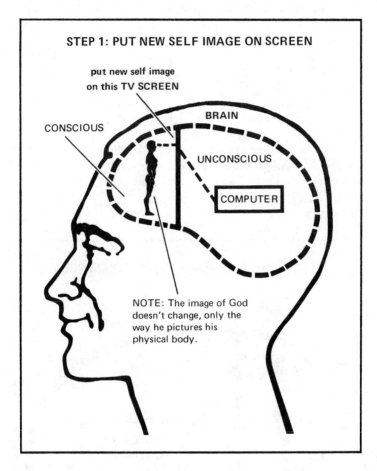

STEP 1: PUT NEW SELF IMAGE ON SCREEN

put new self image
on this TV SCREEN

BRAIN

CONSCIOUS

UNCONSCIOUS

COMPUTER

NOTE: The image of God
doesn't change, only the
way he pictures his
physical body.

Reinforcing Action

To enhance the mental picture, get on the bathroom scale. The dial will come to rest on your present weight. **Ignore that reading.** Reach to the nearby window ledge, towel bar or lavatory counter and press down. This will cause the dial to drop to a lower figure. Press harder until the dial reaches the weight **YOU'D LIKE TO BE**. Hold still for a moment. Stare at the numbers. Think of your eyes as camera lenses. "Click"—take a mental picture of yourself on the scale, weighing exactly that amount.

Forget the fact that you are causing the scale to read this way. Put that out of your mind. From now on— **THIS IS YOUR WEIGHT**—by faith. After this, whenever you think of your weight . . . this is the number you will have in your mind. Etch it into your brain. Remember, God has designed us to do this . . . it's part of the faith process. There's nothing artificial about faith, even when we do things reason cannot explain. Of course this action is explainable. You are simply reinforcing the NEW IMAGE by adding your PROPER WEIGHT to the picture.

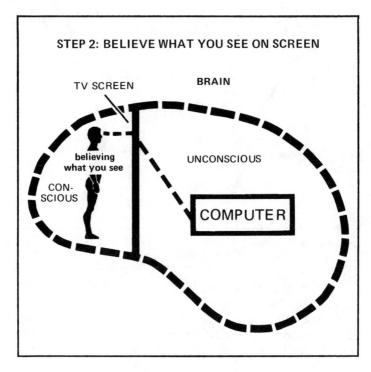

STEP 2: BELIEVE WHAT YOU SEE ON SCREEN

TV SCREEN   BRAIN

believing what you see

UNCONSCIOUS

CON-
SCIOUS

COMPUTER

NOW FOR THE HARD PART

So much for getting the image on the screen. That's the first step. Now for the harder part—**believing it. It is believing what you see that triggers the computer.** It's one thing to SEE yourself as trim and attractive, another to BELIEVE it. If merely seeing the new image activated the computer, we could accomplish all this with day-dreaming or wishing. But wishing doesn't make it so. To make use of the LAW OF BELIEF we have to **believe** what we see on that screen.

ACTION

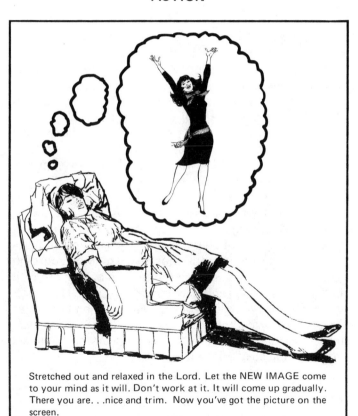

Stretched out and relaxed in the Lord. Let the NEW IMAGE come to your mind as it will. Don't work at it. It will come up gradually. There you are. . .nice and trim. Now you've got the picture on the screen.

Let's say you're a housewife. Your morning chores are finished. You have a moment to yourself. Find that comfortable lounge chair. Stretch out and relax. Let your arms and legs go limp. Close your eyes. Take a few deep breaths and don't do anything. Be still in the presence of the Lord. Then say to Him, **"Lord it feels good to stretch out and relax with you."** That will draw your mind to Him. You're going to be working with Him shortly. Did you not find yourself close to Him during the fast? We want to recapture some of that intimacy as you relax with Him now.

Relaxation

The more you relax, the more effective will be the SEE IT—BELIEVE IT exercise. **Tension binds the imagination.** It's almost impossible to use the imagination as a creative tool when there is tension anywhere in the body. You just can't get clear pictures to appear on your mental screen (the one your computer uses) when you're tense. That's why we don't start dreaming the moment we pile into bed. We have to unwind first. As tension drains from our bodies, the scenes begin to appear in our minds.

Here's how we drain tension out of your system. We start with your right foot. Wiggle the foot and toes so as to become aware of them. Now let it go limp and lazy. Let it sink deeply into the foot rest. Think of your right leg. Let it go limp. Visualize the tension oozing out of it. Let the muscles sag and become dead weight. Now move your mind to your left foot. Wiggle it. Then let it relax. Travel with your mind up your left leg, relaxing every muscle as you go. Now both legs are heavy and limp and lazy, sinking deeply into the chair.

Visualize your stomach muscles. Let them go limp. Don't be in a hurry. Let your mind travel up your back. Become aware of the tension there. Then let everything go limp and loose. Picture the tightness flowing out of those muscles. Shake your head to become aware of your neck muscles. They're tight. Now let them go limp too. Think of them as limp rubber bands with the tension draining away. Become aware of your right arm. Wiggle the fingers. Now let the whole arm go limp. Do the same with your left arm. Take a few deep breaths and then let your head fall limply to one side. Your entire body should feel like a sack of cement. It sinks into the chair as everything goes limp. Picture every bit of tension draining out of your body. Let it sink deeper and deeper into the chair. Every muscle should be relaxed and limp, like loose rubber bands.

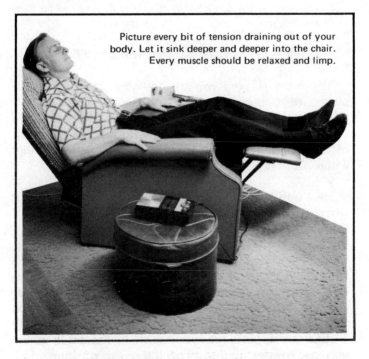

Picture every bit of tension draining out of your body. Let it sink deeper and deeper into the chair. Every muscle should be relaxed and limp.

RELAXATION HELP. The relaxation exercise I described above may not be new to you. Christians today are becoming familiar with some kind of relaxation technique. Note I say relaxation, NOT meditation. This has nothing to do with TM. We live such "hit & run" lives that tensions mount quickly in the course of a day. I am thinking that some of you may have the **HEALING INSTRUCTION CASSETTE** (No. 539) that goes with my book, **JESUS WANTS YOU WELL**. If you do, then by all means make use of it. The same technique applies here. Those of you who are new to any kind of relaxation exercise may need more help than I have given in these pages. If that is true of you, you may wish to take advantage of the **RELAX-ATION CASSETTE** (No. 545) I have prepared for this book. SIDE ONE of this cassette helps you to relax so that your imagination can project a nice trim image on the screen of your mind. SIDE TWO helps you BELIEVE what you see on the screen. It is especially designed to go with this chapter.

NOW YOU CAN VISUALIZE BETTER

The more relaxed you are, the more real will be the scenes in your imagination. Don't go to sleep. This is NOT a hypnotic exercise. I want you alert, thinking clearly, even though your body is relaxed to the point of drowsiness. We want to think through some things while your NEW IMAGE is on the TV screen.

Here and there the Bible speaks of faith as a gift. But what does that mean? It is referring to our **ABILITY TO TRUST GOD for things we don't have as yet—or— to receive from Him things which cannot be seen.** Now the ability to do this is truly a gift. However, DEVELOP-ING this gift, or INCREASING this ability is something else. That's something we do. God doesn't do it for us. I know you have the ability to believe, because God has given it to you. **What I seek to do here is help you DE-VELOP or EXERCISE your faith to the place where you can believe the image on the screen of your mind.**

● One thing that causes faith to rise is being convinced that what you are doing is solidly rooted in the Word of God. Here are three scriptural examples which should

160

establish a firm conviction in your mind:

1. THE CASE OF ABRAHAM

Abraham was asked to believe something **contrary to nature.**

The patriarch was 90 years old and his body no longer able to reproduce seed when God promised him a son. His wife Sarah was barren. Outward circumstances indicated such a thing was impossible. But what did Abraham do? He IGNORED the literal circumstances which said there was no way he could have a son and chose to believe God instead. Fourteen years later Isaac was born (Gen. 15:6; 17:1; 21:5).

To believe that TRIM IMAGE on the screen of your mind, while your body is fat, is certainly contrary to nature. Yet is believing in God's LAWS any more foolish than standing on His PROMISES? The One Who makes good on the promises is the same One Who stands behind the laws—including the Law of Belief; the law we're using in this plan.

2. THE COUNSEL OF THE APOSTLE PAUL

The apostle asks us to SEE OURSELVES in a condition that is contrary to fact.

Did you know the apostle Paul asks us to VISUALIZE a truth that is contrary to the real situation? In the sixth chapter of Romans he asks Christians to RECKON THEMSELVES DEAD TO SIN! (vs. 11). Such reckoning means to COUNT or CONSIDER yourself as sinless! For a Christian, who knows he is a sinner, to reckon himself as "dead to sin," is certainly contrary to the real situation (1st John 1:8). We all sin daily and the Spirit convicts us of it. That's why we're told to confess our sins. We have sinful natures and we sin. True, we also have a holy nature which doesn't sin, but we still choose to sin. Any Christian who thinks he doesn't sin, "deceives himself," says the apostle John.

The apostle Paul knew that if a man pictured himself as a sinner—**and really believed what he saw**—he would sin more and more. On the other hand, if he PICTURED HIMSELF as dead to sin—**and really believed it**—he would sin less and less. Similarly, if a man believes he is FAT, he will STAY FAT. However, if he believes he is TRIM, he will become what he believes about himself. We've learned this is A LAW.

3. THE LOGIC OF JOB

JOB'S faith grew through reasoning.

Job was sorely tested. He lost his health, his wealth, his family and friends. But he was a man of faith, at least SOME faith. As he reasoned and meditated on what he knew of God, his faith began to rise. He worked his way through various reasonings (that's what the book of Job is all about) until he was finally able to utter that grand statement . . . "I know my Redeemer liveth and that He shall stand at the latter day upon the earth" (Job 19:25). His faith was later rewarded with a visit from God in a whirlwind.

If Job could reason his way to faith, **SO CAN YOU.** As you relax in your chair, follow Job's example and work **your** way through the facts concerning the Law of Belief. If you are consistent in your thinking, you'll come step by step to the conclusion that God WANTS you trim and has provided a lawful way for you to BE trim—**by faith.**

● Now put those three scriptural observations together.

Abraham teaches us that we can ACCEPT AS FACT things which are contrary to nature. Paul teaches us that we should VISUALIZE these things to make them true in our own experience. Job teaches us that we can put LOGIC AND LAW together and REASON our way to the necessary faith. Beyond that, Jesus taught us to BELIEVE THAT WE HAVE RECEIVED things even before they are in hand (Mk. 11:24). That's the way faith

162

works. A man doesn't need faith for something he has already received. He needs it for something he doesn't have as yet.

Doesn't it help to realize our program is biblically sound? Sure it does. That brings us to the place where we can start to reason our way to faith. Let's stop here and continue from this point in the next chapter.

SUMMARY

A book is more enjoyable when the truths are broken up into chunks easy to digest. We have bitten off a good chunk this time. Satisfied the **LAW OF BELIEF** is backed by the character and power of God, we have set out to USE IT:

1. We develop a **TRIM NEW IMAGE** on the imagination screen by means of the mirror exercise.

2. We relax our bodies, draining the tension out of them part by part, so that we can project the **NEW IMAGE** onto the TV screen in our minds. Tension in any part of the body hinders the creative use of the imagination.

3. We have checked the Scriptures to make sure our approach is rooted in the Word:

Abraham taught us to IGNORE actual circumstances and trust God for things contrary to fact.

Paul taught us to VISUALIZE the NEW IMAGE.

Job taught us to REASON our way to faith.

Now let's do it. Next.

CHAPTER TEN

Faith Coming Up

"Everything is possible to one who has faith."
(Mark 9:23 NEB)

Did you hear the story of the carpenter hired to work on the night shift of a building project? He was working on a wall several stories high when he lost his balance. As he was tumbling, he managed to grab hold of the edge of the wall. He hung there in the darkness, crying out for help. Other workmen on the job couldn't hear him because of the noise. His cries were drowned in the din of hammers, riveting machines and squeaking cranes. It was pitch black, which added to his desperation.

In time his arms became numb. His fingers ached from clutching. Then he could feel them beginning to let go. Try as he might, he couldn't hold on any longer. He prayed urgently, but there was no miracle. At last his fingers let go. Terror racked his being as he fell—about 3 inches to a safety scaffold that had been there all the time!

164

● Sometimes we Christians are like that. We're afraid to let go and trust God for what He has for us. I'm sure some will feel that way when it comes to dealing with the devil. More will feel that way before going on the fast. And perhaps still more will hesitate to make use of the LAW OF BELIEF. Afterwards though, when they've LET GO . . . to experience what God has for them, they'll rejoice in His wonderful provision.

PRAISE THE LORD, YOU'VE COME THE DIST-ANCE AND ARE IN THE PROCESS OF LEARN-ING HOW TO USE THE LAW OF BELIEF.

I LEFT YOU IN THE CHAIR

We stopped at a convenient point in the last chapter. But we hadn't finished the SECOND STAGE of our **SEE IT—BELIEVE IT** technique. You were just about ready to try reasoning yourself to faith. So let's do that now. You have finished the relaxation exercise. The image is on the screen. You see yourself as trim and at-tractive. It's a nice clear picture. Now to **BELIEVE WHAT YOU SEE,** so as to program the computer.

The following is a check list of steps to faith after the manner of Job:

Place a check mark in the box to the left as soon as you understand each statement and feel the Spirit's witness that it is true.

Since our bodies are temples of the Holy Spirit, we're obliged to keep them trim and attractive for His sake.

☐ However, since the Lord has made it clear that we can't do anything without Him, He must have some kind of help for us.

☐ God's blessings come to us through fixed laws. Inasmuch as everything He does is regulated by His laws (which issue from His nature), we can assume a law exists that we can use in getting rid of fat and maintaining a nice, trim figure.

☐ We have discovered such a law, the **LAW OF BE-LIEF.** By means of this law we are able to make use of the **UNCONSCIOUS COMPUTER** which God has placed in our heads. Since that computer is a substation for the power of God, we know there is more than enough power on hand to help us overcome bad eating habits and control our weight. If we are privileged to use the laws of electricity and gravity and aerodynamics, we know the LAW OF BELIEF is ours to use as well.

☐ From personal experience we already know that ideas **BELIEVED BY THE MIND** affect our bodies. We've all had this happen to us. It's late at night. There's a strange sound. An IDEA races through your mind . . . "A prowler! Someone's trying to break in!" At once you're wide awake. Your heart begins to pound. Adrenalin gushes into your bloodstream. Muscles go tense. Your stomach knots up. Your body is ready for fight or flight.

Then a cat goes, "Meow." You heave a sigh of relief. "It's not a prowler after all. It's just a cat." Then you try going back to sleep. Can you? No. The effect of that IDEA on your body is too great. Here's the point. Even though there was no prowler, YOU BELIEVED THERE WAS. Because you believed an idea that was CONTRARY TO FACT, tremendous forces were unleashed within your body.

Since the body is under the control of the BRAIN, how can IDEAS (which have to do with the mind) affect the body? Ah—the **mind** influences the **brain!** Now that's significant, for the LAW OF BELIEF clearly has to do with the **MIND**. The **brain** can't believe anything. Therefore our bodies can be MANIPULATED by what we believe.

We've all seen this demonstrated by TV hypnotists. Consider the hypnotized subject who is told he's in a steam room. You can watch him break out with perspiration before your very eyes, though he's seated in a chair on stage. Then he's told he's been moved to a walk-in refrigerator. Now watch him shiver and break out with goose bumps. You've seen that, I'm sure. Doesn't it prove that IDEAS do go into the computer, which in turn manifests those ideas in the body? If that weren't so, there'd be no such thing as hypnotism, for hypnotism works with IDEAS only.

Inasmuch as we often PROVE the LAW OF BELIEF in our own experience, should we not accept it as God's will for us, to USE this law for His glory? Since it is scriptural to believe you have something from God BEFORE you actually possess it, we should accept the Lord's counsel in Mk. 11:24 as His instructions to use this law for weight control. It is not only proper to do this, but required since we are stewards of His temple.

NOW THEN—WILL I BELIEVE IT, OR NOT?

That's what you ask yourself as you complete the steps. The program is sound, you're satisfied about that. The LAW OF BELIEF is valid, that's settled. Will you now believe yourself to be trim and slender in advance of the fact? If you will, the NEW IMAGE on the screen of your mind will become a reality. As you weigh the matter, talk to the Lord:

"Lord Jesus, You and I drew closer to each other during the fast. Now You are challenging my faith with the Law of Belief. It's going to take a lot for me to believe I'm thin. But here's what motivates me, Your name is behind Your laws. Therefore trusting in them is the same as trusting in You. Help me to honor You with complete confidence in Your Law of Belief. In the power of Your precious name, I ask You for the faith to be trim and attractive. Thank You, Lord Jesus. Amen."

As you relax in the chair, the Lord is present to every step of your thinking. As you come to the conclusion there is only one way to go, you sense HIS AMEN in your spirit. He knows it's a challenge. But He wants your faith to rise. He can't do the believing for you. All He can do is set the challenge before you and give you His witness. He WILL let you know you are doing exactly what He wants you to do. In fact, it should seem like an ACT OF UNBELIEF not to accept the adventure.

But be assured of this: **God's laws cannot fail.** If you meet the conditions, you will be trim. And you'll agree it is worth the trouble it takes to increase your faith.

HELPING YOUR FAITH ALONG

Now for some more exercises. If your life-style permits, **plan on relaxing in this chair three times a day— morning, noon and night.** The more you do it, the easier it becomes. Pretty soon, you'll find yourself accepting your NEW IMAGE as fact. You WILL believe it. Repetition really pays off. You see, it's all new at first and you're wondering if it will really work. But as the newness passes, doubts are replaced by conviction. So don't think to try it once or twice and then say . . . "It doesn't work." Give yourself time. You'll begin to BELIEVE THAT IMAGE . . . wait and see.

Some daydreaming is called for now. As you relax in your comfortable chair, make MENTAL MOVIES. See yourself in a clothing store buying the enviable sizes. Picture yourself before a full-length mirror, thrilled with the way your new trim sizes fit. That's fun. See yourself coming out of the shop, walking down the street with a spring in your step, a new bounce that attracts attention to your lean look.

Take a mental trip to your doctor's office. Listen to his astounded exclamation . . . "What have you done to yourself? You look absolutely marvelous!" He'll do more than give his usual "hummph," when he finds your blood pressure is 120/80 or lower.

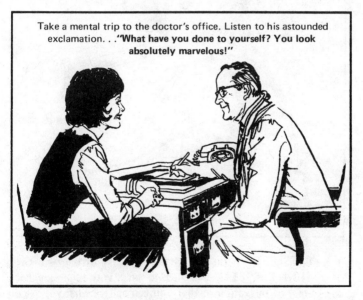

Take a mental trip to the doctor's office. Listen to his astounded exclamation. . ."What have you done to yourself? You look absolutely marvelous!"

You may not be Superman, but you can ride a bike, jump a low fence, dash across a tennis court, send a ball zinging down the bowling alley, romp on the floor with your children or grandchildren. Remember how hard it used to be to get up off the floor? That's gone now. In the movie you're a perfect specimen, full of vigor and vitality. This is the way to THINK THIN. Let your imagination run riot. See yourself enjoying a lithe, supple body. Scenes such as these tend to reinforce your faith in the IMAGE ON THE SCREEN.

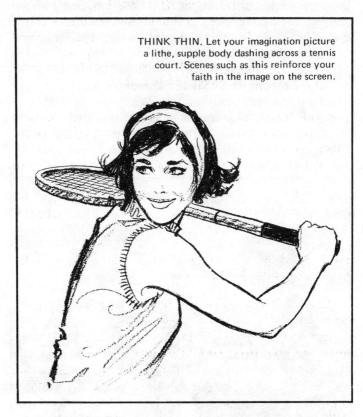

THINK THIN. Let your imagination picture a lithe, supple body dashing across a tennis court. Scenes such as this reinforce your faith in the image on the screen.

CASSETTE. In the last chapter I spoke of the **RELAXATION CASSETTE** designed to help you achieve a deep state of relaxation so that you can believe what you see on the mental screen. Now I want to mention a 3rd cassette, which is perhaps the most important of all, the **NEW IMAGE CASSETTE** (No. 547). It is very different from the other two. It has but ONE MESSAGE, approximately 15 minutes long, repeated 3 times on each side. It is the repetition that finally gets the new image into your computer.

To make full use of this cassette, put the player beside your lounge chair. Make sure the control is within easy reach so that you don't have to disturb your body to operate it. Stretch out and prepare to relax. The more relaxed you are the QUICKER the NEW IMAGE will come alive in your imagination. If you wish to play the **RELAXATION CASSETTE** (No. 545) first, that is fine. The deeper you relax the better. After you achieve a fairly deep relaxed state, remove the **RELAXATION CASSETTE** and insert the **NEW IMAGE CASSETTE** (No. 547).

● The most critical point in your weight control will be when you end the fast and start eating again. That's when you need the most help from your computer. To the degree to which you can get the NEW IMAGE into your computer, to that SAME DEGREE will your computer help you change your eating habits. So you see how vital this cassette can be to your success with this program. Get that new image burning in your imagination and your mind will FORCE you to avoid fattening foods and pass up second helpings. This is far superior to diets or any weight loss plan.

When you have worked with the **NEW IMAGE CAS-SETTE** for four or five days, a NEW YOU will begin to appear on your mental screen spontaneously...with little effort on your part. You'll find that when you pray, the Holy Spirit will bring the NEW IMAGE to mind and you'll begin praising the Lord for what He is doing through your computer. As your faith rises — and it will — your computer will give you more and more help. Therefore working with this cassette puts the success or failure of this plan in your hands. Arrange the exercises to fit your life-style, but do them at least 3 times a day. You won't be sorry.

AT BEDTIME

A prime time for programming your computer is when you're falling asleep. Some people jump into bed

171

and drop off quickly, others not so fast. Whatever the interval, there is a time period when your conscious mind begins to relax its watchfulness. During that period the computer is very receptive to ideas displayed on the screen of your imagination. If you can hold your NEW IMAGE on the mental screen as you are falling asleep, it will affect the computer more positively than at any other time.

You are settling down in bed. You've made yourself comfortable and you're about to say "Goodnight" to the Lord. Just talking to Him while in bed can bring on sleep. As you thank Him for the nice new figure He is giving you, let the new image come up on the screen. Keep it there as long as you can. If you fall asleep visualizing that image, the computer will get the message effectively. Doing this nightly is an important part of the plan.

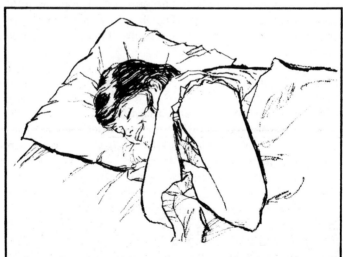

As you thank Jesus for the nice new figure He is giving you, let the new image come up on the screen. Keep it there as long as you can. If you fall asleep visualizing that image, the computer will get the message effectively. Doing this nightly is an important part of the plan.

• Here's a way to get extra mileage out of your **NEW IMAGE CASSETTE** (that is if you have one). It can be a powerful tool at bedtime also. If your player does not have an automatic shutoff, you need a timer. Most hardware stores carry them. They're inexpensive. Get one that will let your cassette run for 45 minutes before it shuts off. Also, pick up a pillow speaker. They're inexpensive too. That way you won't disturb your wife or husband as you play the tape.

Set up the cassette player beside your bed, making sure it is within arms reach so that you can adjust the volume with as little movement of your arm as possible. If you use a timer, set it for 45 minutes. The flat pillow speaker is in place under your pillow. After you say "Goodnight" to the Lord, reach over and turn it on. Hopefully it will continue playing after you fall asleep. Don't try to listen to it. Ignore it if you can and focus on the image on the screen of your mind. Fall asleep as you would normally. Even though you are asleep, the sound will register with the computer. This is why doctors don't allow talking during surgery. People are affected by what they hear when anesthetized. We're exploiting that phenomenon by making it a part of your weight control program. You may find this to be the most powerful element in our approach.

SATAN ISN'T STUPID

What we know, the devil knows. Logic is one of his tools. If **YOU** can reason your way to faith, **HE** can tempt you to reason your way to disbelief. If you listen to him, he'll convince you it is nonsense to believe something contrary to fact. If you don't watch out for him, he'll keep you from using your computer. He knows all about the Law of Belief. The last thing he wants is for your faith to rise to the place where you can **TAP GOD'S POWER** available through that computer. If you are successful in getting the computer to control your weight, then victory in other areas is also possible. That is what he doesn't want.

All along, Satan has had you programmed for OVER-EATING. He isn't going to give up without a fight. You can be sure he will resist every effort you make to put this plan into operation. So get set for an onslaught of negative suggestions. They'll come . . . "How can an intelligent person like you believe he is thin, when his fat is in plain view of everyone? That's ridiculous. The scale doesn't lie." (As if he cared anything about the truth). You'll be bombarded with thoughts such as . . . "If this plan is so great, why didn't God bring it out long ago?" Don't be surprised if members of your own family are among his servants seeking to discourage you.

Remember, the devil wants you fat. He is clever. He's vicious . . . and he'll use every idea and every person he can to keep you from maintaining control over your weight. Now I have warned you. So be alert. Be ready to deal with him. He's out to hurt you, if he can.

SUMMARY

In the last few chapters you've learned some remarkable things. You've learned about your body's computer system and the awesome power it exercises over your body. The SOURCE of its power is God Himself. While there is no way you can reach your computer directly, so as to make it your slave, you can reach it indirectly through the LAW OF BELIEF. In this way, God limits our access to His power to our FAITH. According to the Law of Belief, if you can get the NEW IMAGE on the screen of your imagination and BELIEVE what you see there, your computer will accept it as a COMMAND . . . and seek to reproduce that image in your body.

Bringing yourself to BELIEVE that scene is the big challenge of PHASE THREE of this plan. You have also learned that this approach is completely biblical and that we're working with FIXED LAWS of God. That means there can be **NO FAILURE** if you meet the conditions. The last thing Satan wants is for you to learn how to USE this powerful law to wrest control of different areas of your life from **his hands.** He'll resist you every step of the way, knowing the secret of laying hold of God's power is now in **your hands.**

"Now that I know the law and have an idea how to use it, can't we end our discussion right here and get going?" Is that what you're thinking? Well, the story is not over. Why? If we want the computer to do a job for us, we've got to feed it. How do we do that? By giving it the information it needs to regulate our eating habits. The only way it can get that information is through you. That means you've got to pick up some knowledge about foods . . . so that it can go into your computer. Once it has that knowledge, it will then cause your eating habits to change. It will then compel you to give your body what it needs . . . to look trim and attractive.

That's next.

CHAPTER ELEVEN

Monkeys Don't Have Heart Attacks

"All things are lawful for me, but not all things are profitable. All things are lawful for me, but I will not be mastered by anything."
(1 Cor. 6:12 NASV)

When researchers want to conduct experiments on animals that resemble humans, they use monkeys. If you feed a monkey ordinary monkey fare, he will never have a heart attack. There is no way his body can set up for such an attack on a regular monkey diet. But in 1969 experimenters put a Rhesus monkey on a diet close to that of the average American. It contained 42% fat and about a 50th of an ounce of cholesterol a day.

Within two and a half years, the monkey suffered a massive heart attack. Upon autopsy the heart muscle and coronary arteries looked just like those of a human after a devastating heart attack. That should tell us something of the awful food trap that has been sprung on Americans.

• One of the blessings you will enjoy through computer-controlled weight will be the extension of your life. How come? You will be ELIMINATING from your diet many items that are shortening the lives of millions of Americans. We have a massive health problem in the United States due to the way we eat. While medical science has been successful in bringing to almost zero the number of deaths due to infection, it has been powerless to keep Americans from killing themselves with their knives and forks. We're making great strides in treating various diseases, but we're doing nothing about the real killer—JUNK FOOD.

EATING ISN'T WHAT IT USED TO BE

In earlier days (before 1900) Americans subsisted on a rather simple diet. They raised most of what they ate, securing very few food items from the general store. But that has changed. We don't live close to the soil any more. We live off of grocery shelves. Nearly all of the 15,000 items you find on those shelves are manufactured for TASTE AND LOOKS—not for health.

Here's the situation. Most giant food markets are laid out something like this: Down one side you find the produce. Across the back, the dairy cases and drinks. And up the other side, the meat department. Just about everything surrounded by that U-SHAPED enclosure is **unfit for humans.**

As a result, most of what is sold in our beautiful markets is **NUDE FOOD,** containing little in the way of nutrition, but lots of calories. Maybe someday the packages will be marked: "WARNING: the Surgeon General has determined the contents of this package to be dangerous to your health." Because of the great shift in eating— from the ground to the store—nearly **half** of the American calorie intake **IS FAT!** And of the remainder, one half is sugar. The average yearly consumption of sugar for every man, woman and child in this country is **105 pounds!**

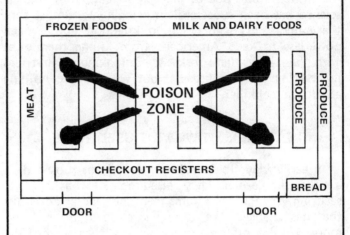

FLOOR PLAN OF
YOUR LOCAL SUPERMARKET

FROZEN FOODS **MILK AND DAIRY FOODS**

MEAT

POISON ZONE

PRODUCE

PRODUCE

CHECKOUT REGISTERS

BREAD

DOOR   **DOOR**

In most supermarkets the only items fit for human consumption are in a giant U around the outer walls. Everything in the middle is poison. Behold row after row of refined products. Once they may have been healthy products from the ground. But now they are cooked and stripped of their nutrition and mixed with chemicals. The vitamins are all but gone. Most of the minerals are missing. The crime is described on the side of the package. It reads . . . "Vitamins A, B, D added." Why? They were all there to begin with. The huge food industry after devitalizing the natural product, puts back a few vitamins so that it can be called a food. If they didn't do that, it would probably have to be sold in a drug store. The industry is getting away with calling it food, but it really isn't. Sugared cereals, for example, should be marked with a skull & cross bones.

NOTE. Most Americans are overweight, but undernourished. The devil has them so locked into sweets and starches, they accumulate mounds of fat on their bodies, while they starve their tissues, blood and vital organs of nutrients needed to function. When the body is overloaded with "food" it can't use, the surplus goes into PERMANENT STORAGE. You are familiar with the common storage areas—hips, buttocks, thighs, waistline, neck and arms, All of it unhealthy.

178

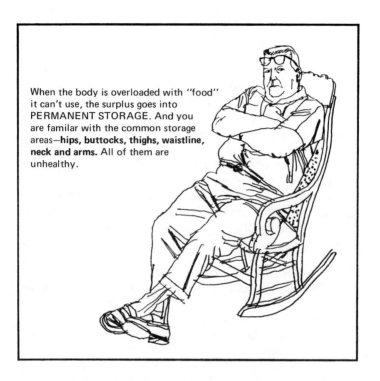

When the body is overloaded with "food" it can't use, the surplus goes into PERMANENT STORAGE. And you are familar with the common storage areas—**hips, buttocks, thighs, waistline, neck and arms.** All of them are unhealthy.

THE BODY PREFERS TO MAKE ITS OWN SUGAR

The body runs on sugar. The various cells function by burning sugar for energy. The body manufactures sugar from the foods we eat; it is programmed to break them down into just the right amount to supply the cells with the sugar they need. But when there is **TOO MUCH** sugar, the excess stays in the bloodstream where it is converted into **FAT.** The only way the body can get too much sugar is for a person to eat too much food or consume sugar manufactured outside his body.

The body likes to make its own sugar, but as you know, it is found in nature and can also be processed from cane and beets. Certain fruits are high in sugar content and honey is practically ALL sugar. So we have to distinguish between that sugar which is manufactured

INSIDE the body and that which comes from an OUT-SIDE source. When you eat anything heavily sugared, a candy bar for example, ALL THE SUGAR in that bar enters the bloodstream **within minutes.** Why? It does not have to be digested. It has already been processed outside the body. As a result, the level of FAT in the blood rises almost immediately.

● For the overweight person whose bloodstream is already loaded with fat, OUTSIDE sugar is a disaster. He must therefore change his attitude toward sugary foods and syrups. And when I say sugared foods I mean everything from cupcakes to sugared cereals. Anything made with sugar should be **OFF LIMITS** for him.

SUGAR. Think of sugar in two forms: SIMPLE CARBO-HYDRATES and COMPLEX CARBOHYDRATES. The simple carbohydrates are table sugar, honey, molasses and syrups. They are composed of few molecules and break down immediately in the body to go gushing into the bloodstream. There they are converted into FAT. Complex carbohydrates, such as potatoes, corn and bread, work differently in the body. When you take a bite of potato, for example, the body must break down the complex molecular structure to convert it into simple sugars. This is a slow process. Sugars converted in this fashion, instead of flooding into the bloodstream, trickle in a little at a time. In this way the body receives plenty of cell energy, but not in amounts that raise the fat level in the blood. If a person is active, and doesn't consume too many carbohydrates, he will burn the sugars as fast as they are manufactured by the body.

Honey and syrups are foods in the same sense that DYNAMITE is fuel. Would a man in his right mind throw dynamite into a furnace instead of coal? Certainly not. Well the person who thinks to run his body on refined sugar is acting with no more wisdom than the man who tries to heat his home with dynamite rather than coal. Coal and dynamite are both fuels.

180

But one burns slowly, giving off steady heat; the other goes off with a bang and is destructive. **What dynamite is to a stove or furnace, sugar is to the human body.**

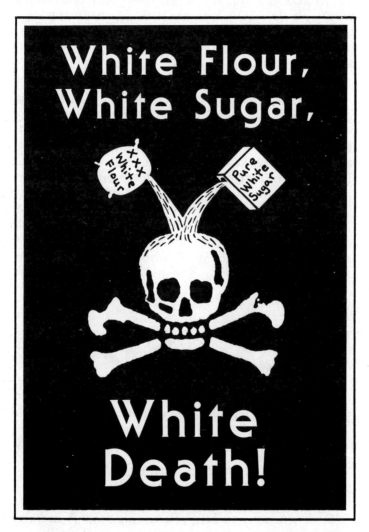

• Wondering about honey? It is a true food. But it is also sugar, a simple carbohydrate. If we were living close to the soil, eating lightly of grains and vegetables and working our bodies to survive, honey would be a blessing. John the Baptist, you recall, lived off of "locusts and wild honey." But in our day, when our bloodstreams are ALREADY LOADED WITH FAT, what was once a blessing is now dangerous. Of all the sugars, though, honey is the most desirable. It contains minerals necessary for good health.

It would be nice to go back to the **NATURAL** eating of years ago, but that is impossible. We can't leap backwards over years of change. But we can definitely control our weight by choosing the best foods available, and avoiding those that contain nothing but calories. In the final analysis, **a man's body is the net product of what he eats and drinks.** The whole business of eating what the body NEEDS rather than what we WANT, is a LAW God has laid down for all animate life. When we get our computers educated as to the foods we should eat . . . and then program them to control our eating habits, we'll see a big difference in both our weight and health.

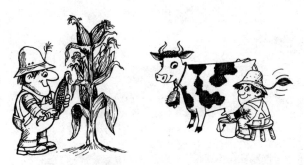

WHAT A FAST TEACHES US ABOUT
FOOD DOMINATION

Once you are on a fast, you quickly become aware of how much your life is dominated by food. While you are fasting, food has NO PLACE in your life. The contrast makes you realize how much of your time was spent in buying food, planning meals, preparing it as well as eating it. When you STOP all that activity, you begin to appreciate the big place food held in your routine. Then, as you continue with the fast, feeling so wonderful with NO FOOD AT ALL, it hits you . . . **"I didn't need all that food I was eating."** If the fast accomplished nothing more than showing you how little food you need to survive, it would be worth the effort.

CRAVINGS. When you learn which foods are harmful, you'll have a new appreciation for the fast. It's hard to give up certain foods once you develop a craving for them, you know, hamburgers, tacos, etc. Normally, it takes anywhere from five to seven weeks of COMPLETE ABSTINENCE from a given food to erase a passion for it. And that's rough for an addict. By means of the fast we cut that time down to about two weeks, plus we break the spell that food has over us. The SHOCK EFFECT of a fast has a destructive influence on a bad habit. Going without ANY food for a period of time makes it a lot easier to give up bad foods while you are programming your computer to take charge of your eating habits. So once more we see the KEY role of the fast in destroying Satan's hold on us through food.

NOTICE

WHAT YOU ARE GOING TO READ NEXT IS FOR YOUR COMPUTER. THE INFORMATION MUST PASS THROUGH YOUR EYES AND INTO YOUR BRAIN TO GET INTO THE COMPUTER. THEREFORE THE FOLLOWING INFORMATION IS NOT FOR COMPLIANCE, BUT TO EDUCATE YOUR COMPUTER. SO DON'T REACT AGAINST WHAT YOU READ. YOUR COMPUTER NEEDS THIS INFORMATION IF IT IS TO ASSUME CONTROL OVER YOUR EATING HABITS.

TRUE FOOD

Food is that substance which the body can convert into energy and use for building cells. Here are items that contain all the nourishment the body needs for any kind of work at any age:

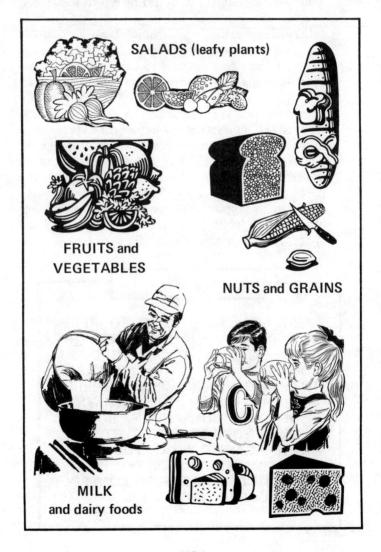

SALADS (leafy plants)

FRUITS and VEGETABLES

NUTS and GRAINS

MILK and dairy foods

The flesh of another animal is not really food in the truest sense, but rather is the RESULT of food. The best meat you can buy has about 30% food value—20% protein and 10% fat. The rest is water. You get better protein from milk, eggs, nuts and grains. However, meat does have Vitamin B12, which is not found in other foods, but is available of course, in your vitamin supplement. Beef should be eaten in small quantities, somewhere around 4 ounces per day. It should be as lean as possible. Then we have poultry and sea foods.

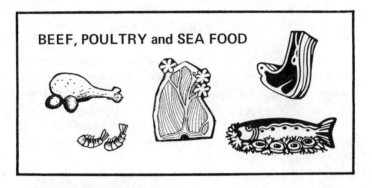

BEEF, POULTRY and SEA FOOD

• There is no way to be a good steward of the Lord's temple and continue eating pizzas, and pastries, ice cream and sweet drinks. Once your computer learns which foods put on FAT, it will move them out of your life. **As God's substation, it has the power to do it.**

This means you must familiarize yourself with **JUNK FOODS** that should be left alone. Such words as calories, protein, carbohydrates and fats will become part of your vocabulary. From now on you should be interested in newspaper and magazine articles that deal with nutrition. The more such information you can feed into your computer, the better job it will do in making you trim and attractive.

MAGAZINES. I'd like to mention two magazines that enjoy wide circulation in the U.S. **PREVENTION** is published monthly by Rodale Press, 33 East Minor St., Emmaus PA 18049. It costs less than a news magazine and gives you an education in nutrition. **LET'S LIVE** is published monthly by Oxford Industries, Post Office Box 74908, Los Angeles, CA 90004. It is full of excellent articles on nutrition. The more you learn about vitamins and minerals and good foods, the better your computer will serve you. It cannot work in the dark. It has to have this information. The only way it can learn it is from you. That means you have to learn about nutrition, so your computer can learn it from you.

THREE SUPER NO NOs

In Chapter Seven I listed some foods to be avoided. I was merely introducing you to the idea there. Now, I'd like to sum up the list of AVOID FOODS with 3 super NO NOs. When you lay hold of the principles behind these 3 no nos, it gives your computer an overall guide in choosing what you should and should not eat. Yes, they take in a lot of territory:

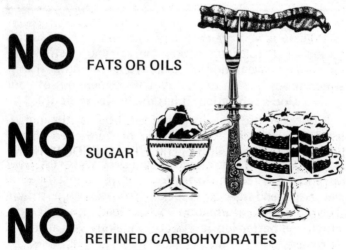

NO FATS OR OILS

NO SUGAR

NO REFINED CARBOHYDRATES

. . . if at all possible, don't even have them in the house.

Good heavens! Aren't you glad this is not for your compliance, but only for your computer! When you consider all the things made with FAT and SUGAR and RE-FINED CARBOHYDRATES it wipes out a host of things we're accustomed to eating. If your computer laid hold of this information and carried it out to the letter, look what would disappear from your life-style:

No more steaks with fat on them, no marbleized prime rib. No cooking oil, salad oil or shortening. Gone would be everything made with sugar, honey, syrup and molasses. Pies and cakes and cookies and crackers would be a thing of the past. Bacon and sausage would vanish, along with whole milk, pickled foods and chocolate. Rich gravies and dressings, ice cream and candy. Everything made with WHITE FLOUR would be gone, along with pancakes, butter and syrup.

Your computer would make a clean sweep of thousands of items currently considered to be good eating. Just think of all the items made with sugar today. Go down the aisle of a supermarket and select any packaged food at random. It will contain sugar. There are about 15,000 grocery products made with sugar, each one on your AVOID LIST. When that news hits your computer, you know your shopping habits are going to be different.

Pick up an ordinary loaf of bread. Look at the ingredients. It might say "wheat flour" or, "enriched flour," but that's to fool you. It's still WHITE FLOUR. If you can find a loaf of bread made with 100% WHOLE WHEAT FLOUR and sweetened with honey, that is about the best you can do—unless you bake your own. As you read these lines, let's advise your computer that everything made with **WHITE SUGAR** and **WHITE FLOUR** is nothing more than **WHITE DEATH.**

Let me repeat, I am NOT offering these NO NOs as something you are to start doing. We simply want the information in your computer. If we get it there and you are successful in programming your computer for the NEW IMAGE, you're going to find yourself looking at these foods differently. In fact, you may smile knowingly as you watch yourself passing up products made with sugars and fats and refined carbohydrates. You'll feel the power of your computer taking charge of your eating habits . . . and you'll thank God that HE gave you such a blessed servant to help you become trim and attractive.

THE COMPUTER SAYS NO

When my granddaughter Jayme was learning to walk, Margie and I had to make a decision about the knick-knacks around our house. We knew the figurines and vases on the end tables would be tempting to little fingers. Should we put them away? Somehow that didn't seem right. We decided she might as well learn some things are OFF LIMITS to Jayme. We left everything as it was.

When Jayme came to our house and would approach one of the delicate items, we'd say . . . "That's a no no." As she'd reach for another, we'd say the same thing. If she decided to touch it anyway, it brought a little slap to the back of her hand. She didn't like that, but it paid off. Before long she was pointing to a vase and saying . . . "No no." Then she'd leave it alone. It was the right way to go. Now we don't have to put anything away when she comes for a visit. We enjoy her so much more.

● This is precisely what your computer is going to do for you. With a little study you can familiarize it with the NO NOs. Then, as you are successful in programming it for the NEW IMAGE, it will gradually assert its power in your life. You'll pick up a package and look at it. From deep within will come a compelling witness . . . **"THAT'S A NO NO."** Your hand won't be slapped, neither will you hear a voice. Yet from within your spirit a powerful rejection will surface. The inner witness will say . . . **"Fat isn't pretty, so put it back. You want to look nice and trim for Jesus."**

Now that's beautiful. You have to fight against yourself to buy that stuff and eat it. And when you do eat it, the pleasure is temporary. You know you have defiled the temple of the Lord, and that's not a nice feeling. A Christian can have guilt feelings over putting a momentary pleasure of the mouth ahead of the Lord's pleasure in his whole body. The more you practice programming the new image, the more powerfully your computer serves as a deterrent.

IT'S NOT ALL NEGATIVE BY ANY MEANS

At our house we have a big toy box for Jayme. While she may not touch certain objects about the place, she has complete freedom when it comes to playing with her toys. In fact, we allow her to scatter her mess all over the living room. She has to pick up everything when she's through, naturally, but she has great liberty otherwise.

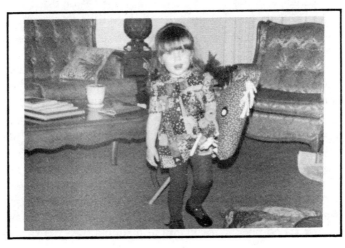

So it is with our new eating habits. WHILE the computer insists we avoid the NO NOs, adventures in good eating await us in the world of fruits and grains and vegetables. When your new taste buds come alive, you're going to luxuriate yourself at the salad bar. Vegetables can be fabulous when steamed. And what's wrong, really, with a small steak, a baked potato plus a chef's salad and diet drink? **If we're going to eat to live, rather than live to eat,** who needs more than that?

Besides, once we break the old cravings, God's power working through the computer is going to create **NEW APPETITES** in us. We'll simply be shifting our tastes from things that make us **fat**, to things that keep us **trim** . . . and enjoy them just as much. The computer will make these changes in us **automatically** when we give it the information it needs and believe the NEW IMAGE on the screen of our imaginations.

WANT TO WATCH YOUR COMPUTER WORK?

I only have space for a few examples, but I thought it would be fun to let you catch a glimpse of how your computer is going to REGULATE your eating once you get it educated and programmed. I could spend a chapter on this alone . . . and you'd love it. But a few situations will let you taste what is coming.

● You're at a buffet offering ALL YOU CAN EAT for a single price. You're moving your tray along the counter. Satan whispers . . . "Yum, yum, doesn't that look delicious? And so does that, and that! It's all yours, as much as you can eat. You want to get your money's worth." Ha! You recognize that voice. Your computer identifies it. You laugh in your spirit as you take note of the few items on your tray and breeze past the dessert section. Satan grinds his teeth. Oh how he hates that computer for giving you such a nice figure.

● You're at the market wheeling your cart past rows of JUNK FOODS. You don't stop. The computer nudges you, "C'mon, let's get to those great tasting fruits and vegetables." You glance toward the packages and jars of processed foods, sensing the terrible reality of Satan's food conspiracy. Praise God He has taken you off the American road to national suicide.

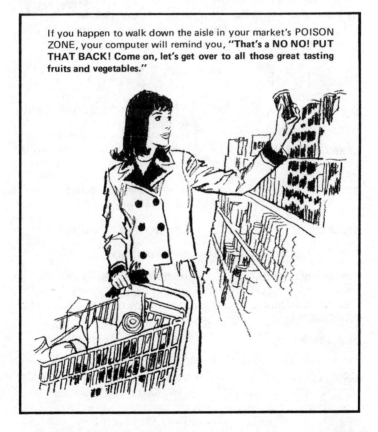

If you happen to walk down the aisle in your market's POISON ZONE, your computer will remind you, **"That's a NO NO! PUT THAT BACK! Come on, let's get over to all those great tasting fruits and vegetables."**

● You find you have X-RAY vision when it comes to choosing what you'll eat. As you look at a piece of pie, for example, you see it for what it is—a glob of refined sugar, white flour, hydrogenated fat, artificial color and a lot of calories. The habit of TURNING ON your X-ray eyes as you look at certain dishes, TURNS YOU OFF to many foods that normally bewitch people because of the way they look. As the computer reminds you what is IN such foods, and what they do to your body, the spell is broken. Thus the computer makes it easy for you to say . . . **"No thank you."**

• You're surprised by the change in your menu. You can see the shift, but you can't believe it takes so little effort on your part. God's power working through the computer is obvious when you note the shift . . .

AWAY FROM	TO*
donuts, pastry, cookies	whole wheat cookies made with honey
bread and rolls	whole wheat bread and rolls (or mixed whole grains)
cereal	whole grain cereals (7 grain, oatmeal, etc.)
crackers	whole wheat crackers
french fries & potato chips	tortilla chips
hamburgers & buns	lean hamburger & whole wheat buns
chocolate	carob
soft drinks	sugar free soft drinks (except cola)
coffee	Postum, Pero, coffee substitutes
tea	herb teas (comfrey, etc.)
pie	custard (rice and honey), pumpkin and honey

*Many of these items are available at your local health food store or health food section of supermarket.

ice cream	honey ice cream or honey yoghurt
spaghetti, macaroni, noodles	whole wheat or vegetable noodles, spaghetti, macaroni
whole milk	raw non-fat (if available)
pizza	non-fat cheese
bacon, ribs, hot dogs, lunch meat	lamb, lean beef, fish, chicken, turkey, eggs
jams & jellies	honey jams & jellies
canned vegetables	fresh leafy vegetables & salads
canned fruit	fresh fruit & melons
salt	onions, garlic, Vege-sal, Spike

● Because your computer is hungry for knowledge about calories, proteins, carbohydrates and fats, you'll find yourself reading books and articles on nutrition. The more you learn, the more powerfully your computer can regulate your weight. Besides, Christian authors like Graham Kerr and Frances Hunter have published books with recipes that are virtually fat free. An exciting new world of **GOOD FOOD** is open to you. Your computer needs that knowledge to make you trim and attractive.

That gives you an idea what to expect. You're going to be thrilled at what happens in your body when your computer begins to regulate your eating habits. You're going to be a new person.

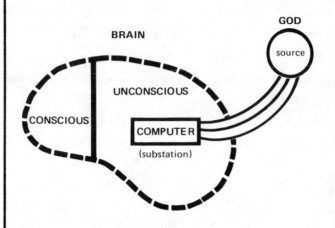

YOUR COMPUTER—GOD'S SUBSTATION

See again the SOURCE of this power to overcome your bad eating habits. It is God's power working through your bio-computer system. Get that computer programmed for the NEW IMAGE and it has more than enough power to do the job. Yes, you can always overrule the computer with your free will. But once you set your heart to please God, you won't want to do that. Rather, you will voluntarily choose to have your eating habits regulated by the computer. Before long GOOD eating habits will be operating in you as powerfully as did the old ones. We all know the power of habits . . . especially if we've tried to break them without some kind of help.

WEIGHT CONTROL—A PERMANENT MATTER

Our bodies will need food until the day they die. That makes eating a PERMANENT proposition. Therefore the only answer to real weight control is a PERMANENT CHANGE in the kinds of foods we eat and the amounts. Such a change seems all but impossible when you consider how the giant food industry has done everything it can to make JUNK FOOD respectable and tempting. When everyone around you is living to eat, it is like swimming upstream to change your eating habits.

Listen to the pain in this letter from a lady who confesses:

"I cannot stop being a glutton! I long to present my body to Jesus as a living sacrifice, but honestly, it is NOT under my control."

That's sad enough, but listen to her PS:

"A woman in our church lost over 100 pounds on Weight Watchers! But she gained it all back in a very short time. Now she's so depressed I'm afraid she may take her life. Isn't there some way we can help her, Dr. Lovett?"

Sure we could help her. I sent information as fast as I could. I knew it would take a lot of POWER to free her from Satan's food trap, but praise God His power is available through the body's computer system. Of course, a person has to know how to use it. That's why I told you **PHASE THREE is the most important part of this plan.** It is using THE LAW OF BELIEF that brings God's help through the computer. And without that help, I don't see any way for a person to make a PERMANENT CHANGE in his eating habits. Now you can see why this plan succeeds where crash diets and fad diets fail.

 Listen to a letter from a lady who has done exactly what I have laid out for you in this book:

"Dr. Lovett, you'll never know what your counsel has done for me. I faithfully followed the plan you gave me and have taken off 60 POUNDS! I'm a new person in Christ! People are coming and asking me to teach this method of weight control in our church. Twenty-five women are now enrolled and they are already losing weight through learning to relax and programming a new image. Twenty-five

more have signed up for a second class. I praise the Lord for leading me to you. I know He is glorifying Himself in what He has done in me!"

(Mrs. R. G. — Minnesota)

SUMMARY

"O, I can't accept Christ, I could never live the Christian life!"

How often do people say that? And how do we reply?

"You don't have to live it. Just let Jesus come into your heart and live His life through you. Little by little He will change you by His own power."

That's precisely what I have been teaching you in this chapter. As you look at the list of foods which MUST go out of your life, you could easily say to me . . . "I could never change my eating habits like that!" Of course you couldn't. **BUT YOUR COMPUTER CAN.** You can no more change your eating habits by yourself than a man can clean up his life without the Lord. You don't have to make the changes, the computer is going to DO IT FOR YOU. That's the whole point of PHASE THREE. That is the exciting hope this book holds out to God's people.

Let me spell it out step by step so there's no mistaking what I'm saying:

1. When a person comes to Christ, he is joined to God. The Spirit of Christ resides within him (Rom. 8:9). This means that the power of God is also present within him. However, God's power is NOT his to use as he sees fit.

2. God's power is administered through the body's computer system. This computer system is already programmed by God to CONTROL the life processes of the body, such as digestion, circulation, maintaining the health and weight of the body. It also

196

functions as a **SUBSTATION for the POWER OF GOD.** This power is both physical and spiritual.

3. Since the computer is located in the UNCONSCIOUS portion of a person's mind, the Christian has NO DIRECT ACCESS to it. That is, he cannot contact it directly or tell it what to do. It is beyond his control. He cannot make it do his will.

4. The only way the computer can be reached, is by the **LAW OF BELIEF.** This is INDIRECT contact. The computer is so constituted that it responds to what a person BELIEVES. Even then it acts according to knowledge stored in it.

5. When a Christian projects a NEW IMAGE of himself onto the screen of his imagination and **BELIEVES THAT IMAGE,** the computer seeks to express that image in his body. It has unlimited power to do this, for it is **God's** power.

6. However the computer must be educated concerning the foods necessary to produce a trim and attractive body. That information is not already on deposit. It has to be learned. The only way it can get that information is for you to learn it and pass it on to the computer. Everything you learn goes into the computer.

7. When the computer has this information, and **YOU BELIEVE** the image on the screen of your mind, it will then go to work to recreate in you a figure as close as possible to the one projected on the screen of your imagination.

8. Satan can hinder the computer by putting doubts in your mind and pressure on your appetite. Therefore it was necessary that you learn how to deal with him. The fast was needed to break his grip on you through the food stronghold. It was the fast that destroyed the devil's power by denying him the very tool he was using against you.

9. The change occurs gradually. As you work with your relaxation and visualization of the NEW IMAGE, the computer will

gradually assume more and more control over your eating. Just as the Lord gradually changes us, so does the computer gradually assume more and more authority. Finally, you'll **AUTOMATICALLY** pass up fattening foods. You'll let the "NO NOs" alone. Then watch the transformation in your body. You'll be like a caterpillar emerging into a butterfly!

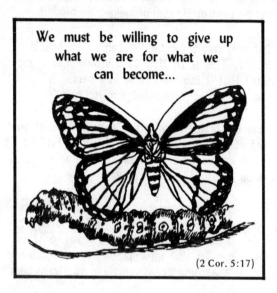

We must be willing to give up what we are for what we can become...

(2 Cor. 5:17)

EXERCISE. At this point, I could easily insert a chapter on exercise. But there's an excellent reason for not doing so—most people WILL NOT do it even though I lay out the steps and show why it is absolutely necessary. For some reason God's people have an aversion to exercise. Therefore it is discussed in a separate book called . . . **JOGGING WITH JESUS**. Those who feel prompted by the Spirit can then have the information they need. Some readers, however, will have copies of my book, **JESUS WANTS YOU WELL**. Chapter Eleven of that book (page 228) deals with exercise. If you have a copy I urge you to read that chapter again. The same principles apply here.

Exercise is vital, not merely because it helps to burn calories, but because it does wonders for the bloodstream, the delivery system of the body. If you can get your heartbeat somewhere between 140-180 beats a minute (depending on your age) and hold it there for about 15 minutes a day, you will open every capillary in your body. Think what it must mean to your brain to have those cells flooded with an abundance of nutrients! Beyond that, exercise is strategic to your weight loss program. It forces your body to produce ENZYMES at a faster rate. For as long as SIX HOURS after you exercise, the increased enzyme activity speeds up the fat-burning process in your body. I'm hoping the Spirit will use these few words to cause you to look into the wonderful world of exercise and what it will do for your body. It can add years to your life.

What I have taught here should be the beginning of your own study to learn more about the foods your body needs. If you'll take the trouble to educate it concerning proteins, carbohydrates, calories and fats, it will bless you beyond words. Notice I haven't told you how to plan your meals. Many weight books offer pages of menus, but I find most people don't pay any attention to them. I will, however, include a **sample diet** or two to give your computer the idea. It is far better for you to become your own nutritionist.

You are now on your way to an exciting new body, one that will attract attention. As the pounds come off, your movements will become more lively. The brilliance will return to your eyes. As you move gracefully and spryly among people displaying your new figure, you'll be a living testimony to what the power of God can do in the believer who wants to present his body to Christ.

Then what? Ah—you can use that glorious new body as a witnessing tool. I think you're going to be surprised to discover how easily a changed body can be used to attract people to Jesus.

That's next.

CHAPTER TWELVE

The Payoff—
For Jesus!

". . .and ye shall be witnesses unto me"
(Acts 1:8 KJV)

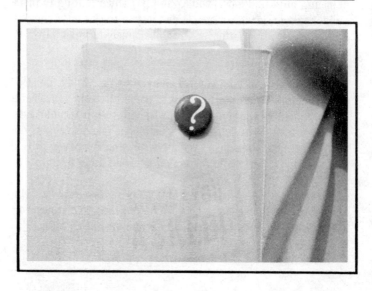

"Brother Lovett, I notice that pin you're wearing. What's it for?"

The man asking the question was the host of a nationwide television show. I had been invited to appear on his national TV broadcast. As I took my place in the big chair provided for guests, I knew my **QUESTION MARK PIN** was conspicuous. You couldn't miss it. It was the first thing he saw.

"I'm glad you noticed my pin."

That's all I said. My hand reached quickly into my shirt pocket. I drew out a tract and offered it to him. He studied it for a second, then laughed . . . "Hey, that's clever!" Then he motioned for the camera to come in for a tight shot. As the tract filled the TV screen, you could see the cover consisted of a great big question mark, matching the one I was wearing. The title stood out in bold type . . . **SINCE YOU ASKED.**

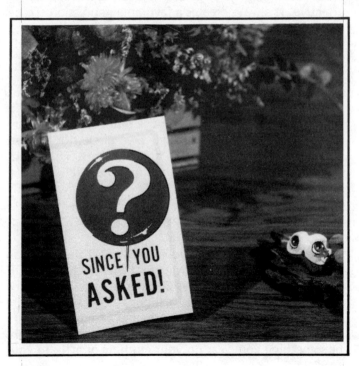

A person wearing such a pin and using a tract to match, doesn't have to **say a word** in order to witness to another person. The prospect sees the pin and asks . . . **"What's that pin for?"** In reply, you simply offer him the tract. When he sees the big red pin on the cover and reads the words **SINCE YOU ASKED,** he knows he has his answer. He gets the connection. Usually the prospect laughs, thinking the joke is on him. Nonetheless you have given him an invitation to Christ, and he doesn't feel you jammed the gospel down his throat.

THIS IS THE PROVOKER CONCEPT

This is a remarkable way to witness. While on the plane travelling to and from North Carolina, passengers and stewardesses alike, asked what the pin was for. All I did was smile and offer each a tract. It was subtle, yet effective. It always creates a favorable impression. To be able to stand in front of a prospect and place the invitation to Christ in his hands **WITHOUT SAYING A WORD** . . . is a neat feat.

A lot of Christians long to speak out for the Lord, but they can't find the words to say. Even if they did, they'd be too shy to blurt them out. As a result, they never say anything for Jesus beyond their own circle of Christian friends. And it goes on like that for years. That's sad. Especially when you consider how easy it is with a **PROVOKER.**

WHAT IS A PROVOKER?

A provoker is anything you use to arrest the attention of a prospect in such a way that **HE INQUIRES OF YOU as to what it means.** Once he speaks to you, the ice is broken. Since HE is making the inquiry, you are not imposing yourself on him by answering his question . . . even though you do it with a tract. A provoker might be something you wear on your clothing or affix to your house or car. The provoker has to be something which is so striking a prospect feels compelled to ask about it. When he does, all you have to do is hand him a tract designed to accompany the provoker.

I'll mention another one to show you what I mean:

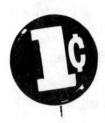

See that pin? When people see it on your lapel, they can't help but be curious about it. Say you're in a restaurant and the waitress sees it. If her curiosity gets the better of her, she'll ask . . . "What does that pin mean?" The reply in this case uses humor, **"You've heard the expression, 'A penny for your thoughts?' Well, I am a THOUGHT-BUYER and I'd give a penny for your thoughts on this . . . !"** Then you offer the tract entitled . . . **A PENNY FOR YOUR THOUGHTS.**

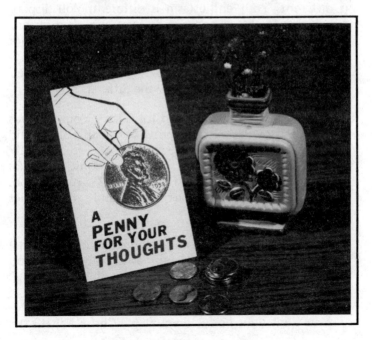

In this type of witnessing, the prospect is the one who INITIATES the action. That's how the Holy Spirit becomes a partner with you. A person who responds to your pin **is someone HE has nudged.** He directs the prospect's attention to your pin and prompts him to ask. When you reply, you are being polite. With this approach you are never blamed for witnessing or accused of being fanatical. The prospect asked and you answered. The usual response is . . . **"That's pretty cute."**

Now why did I take the trouble to explain the provoker concept of witnessing?

YOUR NEW BODY CAN BE A FABULOUS PROVOKER

You've been working with the Lord for a period of weeks now, getting your body into marvelous shape. There's a big difference in the way you look. Your walk is different. Your enthusiasm is different. You display a new zest for life. That trim bouncy body is a far cry from what it used to be. People within your private world will be startled by the BEFORE AND AFTER effect. Those who haven't seen you since you started this program, will be dazzled by the difference.

That difference can be used for Christ. Your glorious new body provides a terrific provoker. People are bound to ask . . . "Wow! What have you done to yourself? You've lost weight, haven't you? You don't seem like the same person! How did you do it?" And so on. Curious friends will be making all kinds of inquiries about your new figure.

Wouldn't it be nice to exploit those comments for the Lord, turning them into a witnessing situation? You can—if **you know how.** Not only will it be satisfying, but it will count for Christ.

You want your body to count for Christ. What's the

point of being trim and attractive unless you're going to use it for Jesus? To have a nice looking body for the sake of appearance only is **vanity.** The Lord Jesus bought us at the price of His blood and He owns us "lock, stock and barrel." We are no longer our own (I Cor. 6:19). The Word instructs us to glorify God in our bodies, but we do the opposite if we doll it up for its own sake. For us to use the Law of Belief to gain nice, trim figures and then not make it count for Him, is the height of self-ishness. The only reason for living, once we're saved, is to honor the Lord Jesus with all we are and have. And to make that nice new body count for Him as we should, means using it as a witness.

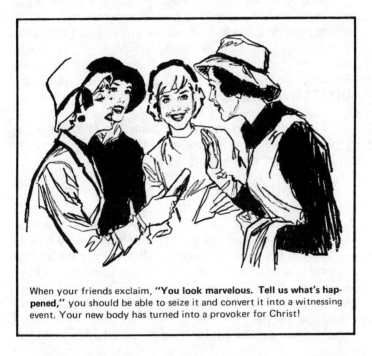

When your friends exclaim, **"You look marvelous. Tell us what's happened,"** you should be able to seize it and convert it into a witnessing event. Your new body has turned into a provoker for Christ!

● Visualize someone who hasn't seen you recently expressing amazement at your new figure. **"You look marvelous. Tell me what's happened!"** That is a golden moment. You should be able to seize it and convert it into a witnessing event. Your body has done its job as a provoker, now it's your turn to exploit the opportunity. Can you picture yourself answering your friend something like this:

"Recently the Lord convicted me that I would look better and feel better if I weighed less. I've tried dieting, but with little success. So this time I asked the Lord to show me how to do it . . . and He did. What you see is the result of working with Him to get my weight off and keep it off. If you'd like to know more about it, I'd be happy to tell you HOW He did it."

Could you say that? I mean, could you come right out with such a statement, boldly and convincingly, to someone you knew only casually . . . and feel at ease in doing it? Or are you saying to yourself . . . "I could never do that!" Now let me ask you something really important . . . **WOULD YOU LIKE TO BE ABLE TO DO IT?** Maybe you're one who says to himself . . .

"I know I should witness for Jesus, but it isn't natural for me like it is for others. I don't think I'm really called to do such a thing?"

OF COURSE YOU'RE CALLED TO WITNESS

I've never met a Christian yet who couldn't witness for Jesus—**if he wanted to.** It's true we all vary greatly in terms of personality strength. What seems easy for one person is a nightmare for another. But there are ways to overcome that variable if a person really wants to witness. For twenty-five years I've been in the business of teaching people how to witness and not once have I found a person who couldn't do it—once he learned how.

The first thing you need to know is this: witnessing and soul-winning are two different things.

When I speak of witnessing, I **DO NOT** mean con-

206

fronting people with Christ and asking them to receive Him as Savior. That's soul-winning. Very few can present Christ to an unsaved person and press him to receive the Lord. That not only takes skill, it takes a great deal of boldness and strength. The average Christian doesn't have the strength for that, at least not at first. But when it comes to letting others know ABOUT Jesus, that is another matter. Any believer can do that—with know-how.

IT HELPS TO SEE THE DIFFERENCE

When I explain the difference between soul-winning and witnessing, you'll agree that witnessing is for you. The idea is not nearly so frightening when you know what is involved. To behold the difference clearly, come with me to a courtroom.

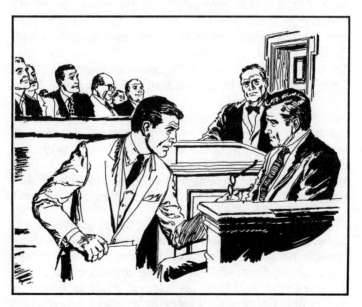

The judge calls the **witness** to the stand. After he's sworn in, he makes statements from his personal knowledge. He is not on trial. He simply tells what he knows.

That's all. He doesn't have to convince anyone of anything. Once he's made his statement, he's all through and steps down. His task is to supply information only. He tells what he knows and that's it.

The **prosecutor**, on the other hand, behaves differently. He doesn't take the stand. He's a lawyer, skilled in handling people, obtaining from them what he wants. Then he uses that information to prove his point. With clever words and techniques he seeks to convince the judge or jury. Everything he does is aimed at getting a decision in his favor.

● **The soul-winner is like a prosecuting attorney.** He employs a skillful approach to the prospect. Using calculated phrases, he extracts information from his prospect and then uses that information to bring him face to face with Christ. With careful timing he moves up to the crisis point and presses for a decision. Everything he does and says is geared to getting his man to DO SOMETHING with Jesus. If he does it right, there is no way for a prospect to avoid a face to face encounter with the Lord. You can see that takes skill and confidence.

Witnessing, is not like that at all. **Once a witness has passed on his information to a prospect, whether by words from his lips or by means of a tract, his work is done.** When believers do not know this, they are inclined to think witnessing means soul-winning. No wonder they panic when someone suggests they witness for the Lord.

Have I said Christians should NOT win souls? No. If a believer has natural gifts that make it easy for him to approach people with persuasive charm, he should be a soul-winner. Such Christians are often salesmen or public workers. Equip them with a systematic approach for presenting Christ and they're instant soul-winners. But for the rest, however, soul-winning is far in the future. They must first START OUT as witnesses to gain the necessary strength and boldness. Later, perhaps, when they have learned to move in the Holy Spirit, and enjoy approaching people for Christ, they could consider soul-winning. But for the moment they should relax in the Lord's words . . . "Ye shall be WITNESSES unto Me" (Acts 1:8).

IT HELPS TO KNOW THIS

I had just finished a soul-winning message in a fundamental church, when a tearful lady rushed forward to speak to me. She was nervous, perspiring. Her hands twisted a knotted handkerchief. She was visibly upset.

"Dr. Lovett, I'm ashamed to say this, but I can't witness for the Lord. I don't know how to win souls. And I'm sure I couldn't do it even if I knew how."

"Forget soul-winning," I said to her. "It has nothing to do with you right now. Why don't you consider becoming a witness. Perhaps later on you can think about winning souls."

At first she was puzzled by my words. Like so many, she thought she couldn't witness for Christ without being a soul-winner. When I explained the difference, her face brightened. Her shoulders dropped in relief. You could see the tension fade from her body. Those few words removed an awful burden from her soul. Then I gave her some easy steps for getting started.

That lady went away rejoicing. As long as she thought witnessing meant she had to WIN SOULS, she was too fear-struck to try anything. The very thought of approaching strangers to confront them with Jesus, made her spirit numb. She knew she couldn't do it. When a person really BELIEVES HE CAN'T DO A THING, his computer accepts it as a command and keeps him from doing it. The Law of Belief was keeping this lady from serving the Lord, because she believed the WRONG thing.

WITNESSING MADE EASY

Earlier I said I had been teaching Christians to witness for more than 25 years. In the process of doing so, the Holy Spirit has developed a unique method for teaching witnessing that works like a ladder. We call it **THE LADDER-METHOD of witnessing.** The ladder has **TEN STEPS** or rungs, with each step a little harder than the last. That way, the Christian learns to witness in bite-sized chunks he can handle comfortably. By means of the ladder, **ANY CHRISTIAN** can become a witness and enjoy it. He starts at the bottom rung and works his way up—**one rung at a time.** He doesn't leave a step until his strengths have developed to the place where he can make the next advance comfortably.

● There are thousands of ways to witness for Jesus, ranging from leaving tracts in secret all the way to telling another person what Jesus will do for him. When a person climbs the ladder slowly, learning to work with the Holy Spirit one step at a time—**witnessing becomes FUN!** Even if it took him a year or more to get to the top, it would be worth it. There's no hurry. In fact, the Lord wants us to **ENJOY** serving Him. When it is fear-filled drudgery, few stay with it for very long.

Now then, isn't that a relaxing truth? Sure it is. So when you start thinking about using your body as a witness for Jesus, don't allow yourself to be terrorized by the notion that you have to buttonhole people and get a decision. Witnessing isn't like that at all. There are easy ways to get started, some of them as simple as leaving a tract in a phone booth, making sure that no one sees you do it. When you realize the Holy Spirit has designed the ten steps to be **FUN,** it should make you eager to learn.

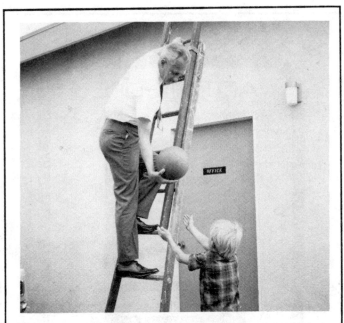

Just as a man cannot go from the ground to the roof of his house without a ladder, neither can a Christian go from silence to active witnessing without a plan which breaks the distance up into easy steps.

GETTING STARTED

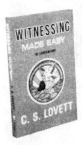

See that book on the left? It's titled **WITNESSING MADE EASY.** It presents the LADDER-METHOD in great detail, showing you how to get started and climb up the ladder one step at a time. On the first two rungs, you have NO contact with people at all. This means there is no interpersonal threat. You begin by leaving tracts secretly. They have to be secret because you will be conducting experiments with the Holy Spirit to sample His power.

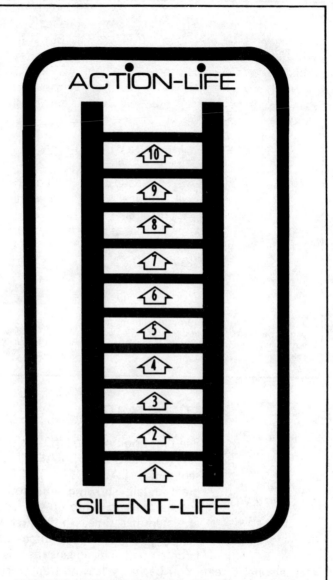

BECOMING A WITNESS IS EASIER—ONE STEP AT A TIME.

The first thing you learn in this approach is that it is the Spirit of God Who makes witnessing easy. I know you agree with that idea IN THEORY. But wait until you meet it in PRACTICE! Wow! I assure you it is thrilling to experience His power IN AN ACTION STEP. When you see how the Holy Spirit calms the flutters in your heart, you'll kick yourself for not getting started sooner.

NOW FOR SOME ENCOURAGEMENT

It's one thing for me to speak of the thrill of the witness-life, another for you to hear it from someone who started from where you probably are right now. Listen to the testimony of this dear brother who went up the witnessing ladder. I have his permission to use his letter, as well as permission to use other letters you'll read:

> *"My life started to change with the third lesson. It has continued to change as I made my way up the ladder. I have found great enjoyment in working with the Holy Spirit and seeing Him work through me. I have grown from an inactive Christian to a bold witness. I have little fear and I do not allow anything to interfere with a witness situation. I now know for a fact that the Holy Spirit supports a person from the very first move he makes. I feel the Lord can now use me anywhere, not only because of the know-how I have acquired, but because I know how to listen to the voice of the Holy Spirit. I could never go back to the life of a routine Christian."*

(Eugene Walters, St. Marys, OH)

Isn't that something? I have boxes of letters like that from people who were once timid and shy, thinking they could never witness for the Lord. But when you USE A LADDER, even the feeblest saint can go the distance—**one step at a time.** Should you hear a voice from within

213

saying, "You can't witness, you're not made that way," or, "You're not called to witness," you can be sure it is not your heart saying those words, but Satan. He doesn't want you to have the joy of witnessing for Jesus, so he plants those ideas in your mind. Take my word for it . . . somewhere on the witnessing ladder IS A LEVEL where you **can witness comfortably.**

Still feel uneasy about the idea? Listen to this:

> *"Before I read this book, I was afraid even to let others know that I was a Christian. I would turn red if someone asked me to say something about the Lord. But now that I have completed each step of the ladder, I have the confidence to speak out for the Lord in any kind of situation. I have learned that the Holy Spirit really does speak through us."*

(Martin Freust, Downey, CA)

See why I say YOU CAN use your body as a provoker? It is possible for a SHY, TIMID Christian to gain the boldness he needs, no matter how scared he is of others when he first starts out. If you learn the words to say (not many of them either) and how to handle yourself in the witnessing situation, the Holy Spirit will take it from there. It's easy . . . **when you know how.** It has been my joy to work with thousands of Christians who echo these testimonies.

● Think how great it is going to be to honor the Lord for the miracle He has produced in your body! You'll be able to say with Pat Vickers, Julian, WV . . . *"What a marvelous world has been opened to me through this method of witnessing. Now my conscience is clear concerning the Great Commission! Praise God!"* What joy to have a clear conscience with regard to the one command the Lord gave us all. I'm sure you want that. Well, you can have it. In fact, once you get started, you will

214

find yourself caught up in the thrill of exalting Christ. Here's a housewife who "stumbled" into the excitement of witnessing for the Lord:

> *"This book has transformed me into an outspoken and bold Christian. Once I was afraid of what others would think if I spoke to them about Jesus. Now I thrill to letting the Holy Spirit do it through me every chance I get. I am so grateful I 'stumbled' onto this book. Each day is so exciting and full of joy. I don't want to do anything but serve Him all the days of my life. I can't begin to find the words to describe all the glorious things that have happened to me since I learned to witness this way. Right now I'm weeping with joy! Praise the Lord!"*

(Cindy Goss, Jacksonville, IL)

● Did you know our bodies respond to the exhilaration of witnessing? When you sense you are honoring the Lord, contentment saturates your being. There is no worse feeling for a Christian than to think he is failing his Master. And no richer feeling than to sense he is pleasing the Lord. When the Spirit uses you in power, deep satisfaction floods your soul. The fun and enthusiasm which go with Spirit-filled witnessing put new bounce in your body. You become a different person. Listen to how Roger's life was changed through witnessing:

> *"I am having the thrill of a lifetime WITNESSING for Jesus! I never dreamed it would be this way! From what I have tasted already, I know I have to be a witness for the rest of my life. Thank you, Brother Lovett, for your wonderful book and the help it has given me. My life has changed completely! I am a TRANSFORMED MAN ALL OVER! Witnessing for Jesus is the one big adventure of this life!"*

(Roger E. Duperree, Punxsutawney, PA)

All those exclamation marks in that letter are his, not mine. You can tell he was having a hard time finding words to describe the thrills that go with the witness-life.

How about it? Are you ready to present that nice, new body to the Lord and let HIM use it as a provoker? It's yours now. You wrenched it away from Satan via the fast. You can give it to Jesus now. I trust you will. Take my word, once you learn how to witness in the power of the Holy Spirit, you can have a lot of fun with that new figure.

COME ON, TAKE THAT STEP

In the back of this book you'll find a list of the titles mentioned in this book, among them **WITNESSING MADE EASY**. Before Satan has a chance to pour cold water on your spirit, why not go to your desk right now and get off an order? Yes, you could go to your bookstore and that might be faster, but it would mean a lot to me if you were to drop me a note saying,

"Dear Dr. Lovett, I want to use my new body for the Lord Jesus. I sense the Spirit's call to be a witness for Him. If you have a plan for helping believers witness at their shyness level and easing up the ladder, I'm interested. Please send me a copy of **Witnessing Made Easy** and bill me for it. Thanks for helping us give our best to the Lord."

In His precious name,

Signed _____

Address _____

City _____

State, Zip _____

Questions Frequently Asked

AFTER READING THIS BOOK

---

1. QUESTION: "I'm too nervous to fast. I've tried it and I become weak, irritable and hard to live with. Is there something else I can do?"

ANSWER: Bear in mind the Lord designed our bodies for fasting. Fasting is HIS idea, not ours. But we're not all alike. So if fasting makes you nervous, you can overcome this by EASING INTO IT. Start by missing one meal a day on a regular basis. Do this for a week or so. As soon as you can handle that, try going without food from Saturday night to Monday noon. When that becomes manageable, try a two or three day fast. Before too many weeks go by, you should be able to start a ten day fast.

COMMENT: There are FIRST TIME FEARS connected with fasting. Fear of fasting can do much to hinder you.

This is why so many have to fast more than once to achieve the desired results. Some are not really comfortable until their second or third fast. They have to DISCOVER FOR THEMSELVES that fasting won't hurt them. Once they make this discovery, the fear vanishes and many disagreeable symptoms disappear.

2. QUESTION: "What can diabetics or hypoglycemics do about fasting?"

ANSWER: Unless a diabetic is under a doctor's care, he should not attempt to fast. Unless his doctor is willing to watch over him and keep him out of trouble, it would be unwise for him to attempt fasting on his own. However, some borderline diabetics do fast successfully. I have received letters from diabetics and hypoglycemics (those with low blood sugar) who have successfully completed the ten day fast. Some even told me their condition was improved by the fast.

COMMENT: One day fasts can be very beneficial. They will NOT break Satan's hold, but they provide a discipline that, in time, helps you get a handle on your appetite. If your diabetic condition will tolerate a one day fast, pick out the best day of the week for you, and stay with it for a time. I think you'll be pleased with the results. You may even graduate to a three day fast. As you may know, hypoglycemics can manage quite well by eating the right kinds of foods at the right times.

3. QUESTION: "When I went on the fast, I got so weak and hungry I couldn't stand it. I hated breaking the fast, but I had to. Any hints that would allow me to continue the fast?"

ANSWER: Rather than have you break your fast early, I suggest you brew an 8 oz. cup of herb tea (any flavor you like), add ¼ teaspoon of honey and the juice of ¼ lemon. Sip the mixture slowly — only as you need it. The honey (already digested by the bees) will go directly into your blood stream to give an energy boost. The lemon will perk up your liver and the tea has medicinal value. If you had to do this every 3 or 4 hours to get you through the hunger (weakness) interval, it wouldn't interrupt your fast. There is not enough carbohydrate present to activate your digestive system.

> **NOTE:** If this does not give the help you need, purchase a bottle of **STEERO** (5½ oz.) at the market. It costs around 50¢. Stir a ¼ teaspoon into a cup of hot water. Use it as above. If that doesn't work, you may have to shift from using nothing but water, to **DILUTED** vegetable juice. Fruit juices are high in sugar. Make up a supply and keep it in the refrigerator. But be tough on yourself and try and get by with as little as possible. Dilute half water with half juice.

4. QUESTION: "I suffered severe heart-burn during my fast. Is there anything I can take to ease the distress?"

ANSWER: Some have told me that using an antacid does not interfere with the fast. Di-gel is a product that seems to work fairly well.

5. QUESTION: "Should one continue taking vitamins while fasting?"

ANSWER: Vitamins are used in connection with food. They are useful in getting the most out of what you eat. But if you eat no food, nothing is gained from taking them. The fact is, a normal body provides itself with a hidden store of nutritive materials concealed in such places as bone marrow. Unless you were planning on going on an extended fast, there really is no need to take anything but water.

> **COMMENT:** If you are one who has to use the herb tea and honey to get through the weakness period, there would

be no harm in adding ¼ teaspoon (1,000 milligrams) of **crystalline** Vitamin "C" to each cup. I like comfrey tea, which is but one of the many herb teas sold in health food stores.

6. QUESTION: "I went on the fast. Everything worked as you said it would and I lost a lot of weight. But since I have started eating again, the weight is returning so fast, I'm scared. What should I do?"

ANSWER: When your weight zooms back up not long after you've come off the fast, it means the APPETITE HAS NOT BEEN CONQUERED. What do you do? Plan on another 10 day fast a month later. Many readers have found it necessary to fast three and four times before they finally gain complete control over their eating. ALSO it means the NEW IMAGE has not been burned into your mind. Likely you are not making sufficient use of the **NEW IMAGE CASSETTE.**

NOTE: Once you get the weight off, you'll be surprised how little food it takes to hold your weight. We all eat far more than we need. So set a FIVE POUND limit on the amount you'll allow yourself to gain back, saying, "BEYOND THIS I WILL NOT GO." When you reach that limit, STOP EATING AT ONCE. Do not eat again until your weight is back where it was when you ended your fast. Usually a day or two is sufficient. Some find they have to fast one day a week to keep their weight where they want it.

7. QUESTION: "Is it all right to take aspirin while fasting?"

ANSWER: Those who are used to drinking coffee and have to give it up to fast, can suffer withdrawal headaches. Others can have headaches too. But as to taking aspirin, that is possibly a medical question. Since I am NOT a medical doctor, I can only pass along what other researchers have found. When you fast, medicines and drugs are many times more POTENT than when you are eating food. If you must take them, the researchers suggest you cut your dosages way down. Actually, if your doctor agrees, it is better to eliminate them entirely. If you elect to experiment on your own, start off with tiny amounts. With no food in your system, it won't take much to aleviate the pain.

8. QUESTION: "After I fasted four days, I had so much nausea and pain, I had to quit. Does this mean fasting is not for me?"

ANSWER: You were correct in stopping the fast. But please remember how I told you in the book, that you can expect almost anything from a pain in your hip to a toothache. There can be heart-burn, nausea and cramps, as well as headaches. Your body is going to object to going without food. Since your doctor has already cleared you for the fast, you know these symptoms are nothing more than your SPOILED BRAT kicking up a fuss. Don't get discouraged. The next time you try the fast, you'll be more relaxed. The more relaxed you are, the less distress there is.

> **COMMENT:** Many of the aches and pains are due to tension and fears in connection with fasting. Symptoms which you would ordinarily ignore, are intensified by fear. When you are worried, they multiply and become exaggerated. It's something like when you are left alone at night. You hear every sound in the house. In the daytime you don't think anything about them. So it is with every little ache and pain that accompanies fasting. You wonder if you're hurting yourself. But God would never ask us to fast, if He knew it would hurt us. Once you discover how normal fasting is, you'll relax. When you do, the symptoms will become far less bothersome.

9. QUESTION: "My husband is unsaved. He wouldn't

understand fasting. Is there any way I should work around him?"

ANSWER: Don't try. When he's in a good mood, mention to him that you would like to give him a trim and attractive wife...because he deserves one. Explain you can do this by going on a fast, and that you'd be willing to do it for his sake. You can ease his mind by assuring him, it will not in any way affect the meals you fix for him. Any man in his right mind wants a trim and attractive wife at his side.

COMMENT: It will be tough fixing 3 meals a day for a man (family) while you are fasting. But if you make good use of the **"GETTING OVER THE HUMP" CASSETTE,** you'll pass through the hunger period. After that, it won't bother you nearly as much. In this situation you may have to rely more on the tea and honey. **Caution:** When you speak of fasting to your husband, DO NOT mention the spiritual side of fasting. You want your mate to think it is all for him. In your heart, of course, you will actually be doing the fast with the Lord Jesus...and for HIS sake.

10. QUESTION: "I'm pregnant. Should I fast?"

ANSWER: Many pregnant women suffer "morning sickness" as it is called. This is simply the body seeking to rid itself of toxins in preparation for the new baby. Sometimes there is vomiting and loss of appetite. The body wants no food. This would be an ideal time for a pregnant woman to go on the ten day fast. She should begin when she feels the first faint start of nausea and vomiting. Ten days of fasting would put her body in great shape for her baby. There should be no morning sickness after that.

COMMENT: If nursing mothers fast, they should know that fasting will stir up toxins in the body and could go to the baby. For this reason, some authors recommend the mother put her baby on a bottle for the first 4 days of fasting. After that, she can resume breast feeding.

11. QUESTION: "Is there any harm in chewing gum while fasting?"

ANSWER: Make it sugarless, such as Trident, and you won't have any trouble.

12. QUESTION: "It wasn't until the 10th day that I enjoyed any dramatic closeness to the Lord. Is this normal?"

ANSWER: The first time you fast, your mind is occupied with fears that you might hurt your body. The next time you fast, you'll be far more relaxed and should become spiritually sensitive about the 7th day. Some have told me they do not reach the spiritual state on their first fast, but enter it easily on subsequent fasts. This might be true of you.

13. QUESTION: "I've noticed the cassettes you offer with the book. How important are they? Do I really need them?"

ANSWER: A person can read the book and take off the desired weight, but that is not the objective. It is PERMANENT weight control you want. Unless you re-program yourself for a NEW ATTITUDE toward food, any weight you take off will NOT STAY OFF. You must get your body's computer system programmed for the NEW IMAGE. And that's where the cassettes become important. They help get the NEW IMAGE into your computer. Once that happens, this powerful bit of mental machinery will work WITH YOU to keep your body trim and attractive. But without that kind of programming, you'll find your own body FIGHTING AGAINST YOU. For permanent success, you may have to fast more than once and make systematic use of the cassettes, particularly the **NEW IMAGE CASSETTE**.

14. QUESTION: "Since this approach is so effective in weight control, couldn't it also be used to deliver Christians from smoking and drinking habits?"

ANSWER: Indeed. The same principles can be applied to almost any addiction, even drugs and self-control. But one must recognize the principles and be able to apply them. If you are one who can do this, then go a-head and try. You have nothing to lose but your problem. As the Lord leads, I may be doing this for you... preparing cassettes for specific habits such as smoking, drinking and temper control.

> **NOTE:** Some have written complaining they are not gaining positive control over their appetites. Yet their letters make no mention of looking to the Lord for help. Let me affirm again — this is HIS approach to a trim and attractive figure, not mine. In my judgment there is no way to use this approach successfully apart from Him. So if you are not getting the results you desire, it could be wise to check and see if you are really doing this with Jesus, or simply trying to do it on your own. If you leave the Lord out of your program, you may well find it IMPOSSIBLE to gain positive and complete control of your appetite. He made it very clear...

"Without Me ye can do nothing" (John 15:5).

Sample Diets

AND BRAN DISCUSSION

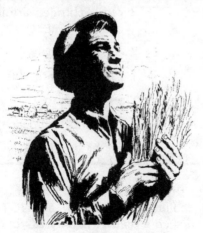

   While few people pay much attention to the pages of receipes included in most books on weight loss, you do need a rough idea of what's involved. Here are a couple of diets for one day:

DIET NUMBER ONE

BREAKFAST:
- ½ cup unsweetened orange juice
- 1 egg, soft boiled or poached
- 1 slice whole wheat toast
- ¼ cup grape-nuts cereal
- 1 cup non-fat milk

LUNCH:
- 2 ounces broiled chicken
- ½ baked potato
- ½ cup (about 4 oz.) cooked vegetable, squash perhaps
- 1 teaspoon margarine
- ½ cantaloupe

DINNER:
- 3 ounces broiled sirloin steak
- ½ cup diced beets
- 1 teaspoon margarine
- 1 small tomato
- 1 medium fresh peach

Be sure to supplement your diet with good vitamin and mineral tablets. Remember, I am NOT TELLING you to go on such a diet. It is only as your computer, armed with this information, empowers you to enjoy such a diet that you will eat in this fashion. If you have to force yourself to eat this type of meal, it will never become a permanent part of your life style. So again, this information is for your computer only, that it might assist in your reduced food intake. Now here's another:

DIET NUMBER TWO

BREAKFAST:
- 1 whole orange
- 2 oz. meat, fish or fowl
- 1 piece whole grain toast
- 8 oz. non-fat milk

LUNCH:
- 4 oz. meat, fish or fowl
- 4 oz. of vegetable (beets, broccoli, cauliflower, tomatoes, string beans, cabbage, or mushrooms)
- 1 piece of fruit
- herb tea or diet drink

DINNER:
- ½ glass tomato juice
- 4 oz. broiled sirloin steak
- ½ baked potato
- 1 teaspoon margarine
- lettuce hearts salad, low cal dressing
- diet drink
- ½ cup water packed fruit salad or a medium sized apple

Allowed fresh fruit: oranges, apricots, grapefruit, peaches, pears, or pineapple.

WHAT ABOUT BRAN?

Bran is making news in the nutrition world. Dr. Rubin's *SAVE YOUR LIFE DIET*, has caused many to experiment with it. When you start eating again, after you have achieved your desired weight, it would be a good idea to include bran in your diet. It's cheap, costing about 70¢ per pound. Dr. Rubin says that 6 teaspoons a day will spare you a host of problems in your body. I have found this to be so.

If you find you CANNOT get a lot of unrefined foods on your table, you can boost your fibre intake dramatically by adding unprocessed bran to your program. You can forget the calories, for bran causes you to excrete fat. And if you are one who is bothered by either constipation or diverticulosis or a spastic colon, you could find yourself praising the Lord for a miracle.

Make sure, however, that you get **unprocessed** bran. That is bran that has not been turned into some kind of breakfast cereal. The bran you want comes straight from the mills where it has been separated from the wheat berry. Health food stores carry it and it is also available from mail-order vitamin houses. If you got only a couple of tablespoons into your diet each day, the results would be very noticeable and the cost negligible.

> **HINT.** Bran tastes like sawdust. You can't put a spoonful in your mouth and swallow it. It's too dry. I have conditioned myself to put a teaspoonful in my mouth and flush it down with water. I use 3 tablespoons a day for my own needs. It's fantastic for constipation. If you mix yourself a protein drink for breakfast, you could add a couple of teaspoons of bran and it would go down easily. If you bake, about ½ a cup to 4 cups of flour is about right. You can add it to soups, gravies or mix it with your breakfast cereal. You can even sprinkle it on salads or mix it with meat loaves. The quickest and easiest way for me is to wash it down with some liquid.

• A doctor Sanford Siegal of Florida, director of 10 obesity clinics, puts his patients on NINE TABLE-SPOONS of bran a day and then tells them they can eat almost anything they want . . . and they'll lose weight. After they take off their excess weight, he still keeps them on the 9 tablespoons of bran. He calls this a "permanent weight loss diet."

Note he says they can eat ALMOST anything they want. "To lose weight," adds Dr. Siegal, "you must eliminate all refined carbohydrates, especially sugars and white flour from your diet . . ." That sounds familiar doesn't it? He advises his patients to use artificial sweeteners and whole wheat flour. Do that he says, "and you can eat anything else you want."

NOTE. If you're tempted to experiment with Dr. Siegal's bran approach, he advises starting with ONE TEASPOON three times a day. You have to build up to the 9 tablespoons gradually to avoid cramps and diarrhea. If it makes you gassy, he says, it subsides in a few weeks. Another physician explains how it works: the swift movement of the bran through the body provides less time for energy to be extracted from foods. This also means that cancer producing agents have less time to do their dirty work. Dr. Siegal's plan is backed by Drs. Emanuel Cheraskin, of the University of Alabama and Olaf Mickelsen, professor of nutrition at Michigan State University. They affirm that such an eating program not only can prevent heart disease, gallstones, hemorrhoids, and blood clots, but cancer of the colon as well.

WHAT ABOUT VITAMINS?

"You leave it up to us to learn about vitamins and minerals. But when a person starts reading the literature on this subject, it is a little bewildering. Could you give some idea as to how a person should get started?"

Below you will find the daily supplements suggested by Dr. Paavo Airola, Ph.D., N.D. (a frequent writer in **LET'S LIVE**) as a beginning point. You will no doubt make your own changes in his approach as you learn more about vitamins and the type of stress you live under. But at least it does provide a starting guide:

1. **Vitamin A** . . . . 25,000 I.U. made from fish liver oil.

2. **Vitamin E** . . . . 100 to 600 I.U. Mixed tocopherals from vegetable sources.

3. **Vitamin C** . . . . 1500 to 2000 mg. (I use ascorbic acid, it's much cheaper.)

4. **B-complex** . . . . . . high potency with B-12 (from yeast.)

5. **Bone meal and kelp for minerals.**

   HINT. You can write to **LET'S LIVE** magazine for a copy of Dr. Airola's article . . . "Are vitamins and food supplements really necessary?" It will give you a quick overview of the field, with a little discussion on each of the important vitamins. The article appeared in the JULY 1977 issue, and you can contact the magazine at Post Office Box 74908, Los Angeles, CA 90004. I suggest that you subscribe to **LET'S LIVE.** Over a period of time it will give you an education in health.

HOW ABOUT VITAMIN OVERDOSES?

Now and then you hear of isolated cases where some-one has foolishly taken a tremendous overdose of vita-mins and suffered a toxic reaction. Then the news servic-es pick up the story and make a big issue of it. The truth is, you can even poison yourself with GOOD FOOD if you eat too much of it. If you were to ask, "Is it possible to take too many vitamins?" the answer, according to the prestigious **Merck Manual,** is that it would take any-where from 600 to 60,000 times the amount required for optimal nutrition.

Consider Vitamin A for example. Dr. Airola suggests a minimum of 25,000 units a day. And he has been do-ing this for years with nothing but good results. The **Merck Manual** says that the average adult can tolerate doses of 300,000 units daily. The same manual goes on to list SAFE DOSES. Here are some examples that will show how harmless vitamins really are. These are the UPPER LIMITS for daily adult doses:

Vitamin A . . . . 300,000 units

Vitamin D . . . . 80,000 units

Vitamin B-1 (Thiamine)   2,500 mgs.

Vitamin B-2 (Riboflavin) 6,000 mgs.

Niacin (Niacinamide) . . . 5,000 mgs.

Vitamin C (ascorbic acid) 15,000 mgs.

From these figures it doesn't seem likely a person is going to poison himself with vitamins unless he wants to start swallowing about 600 tablets or more a day. A person in his right mind wouldn't do that. You wouldn't do that. You wouldn't surely.

THE "BASIC FOUR"
FOOD GROUPS

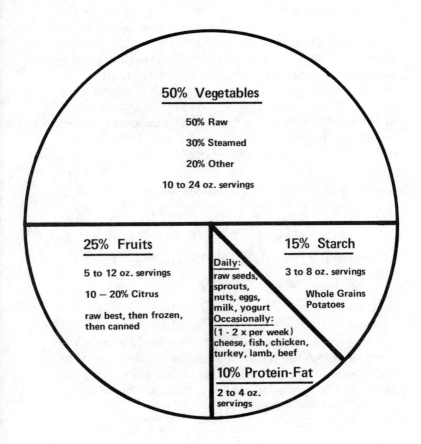

50% Vegetables

50% Raw

30% Steamed

20% Other

10 to 24 oz. servings

25% Fruits

5 to 12 oz. servings

10 – 20% Citrus

raw best, then frozen,
then canned

Daily:
raw seeds,
sprouts,
nuts, eggs,
milk, yogurt
Occasionally:
(1 - 2 x per week)
cheese, fish, chicken,
turkey, lamb, beef

10% Protein-Fat

2 to 4 oz.
servings

15% Starch

3 to 8 oz. servings

Whole Grains
Potatoes

LIVE LONGER AND BETTER DIET PLAN

Rather than a menu, this will give you a broader base for designing your own meals. If you wish to eat protein first, that is all right. The daily requirements are shown in ounces. Don't feel bound legalistically, but use these figures as a general guide. You really need some sort of a guideline and this can provide it.

Foods Allowed

50% Vegetables - 10 - 24 Oz. daily requirement.
50% raw; 30% steamed; 20% other, i.e. baked, etc.

3% Natural Sugar

Asparagus
Beet Greens
Broccoli
Cabbage
Cauliflower
Celery
Cucumber
Endive
Eggplant
Green Pepper
Lettuce
Mushrooms
Okra
Radishes
Sauerkraut
Spinach
Tomato

6% Natural Sugar

Beets
Brussel Sprouts
Carrots
Green Beans
Kohlrabi
Onion
Pumpkin
Rutabaga
Squash
Turnip

Try these raw with dip made of avocado, garlic, onion, and lemon juice, or cream cheese, onion, lemon juice and paprika.

15% Natural Sugar

Artichokes
Green Peas
Parsnips

20% Natural Sugar

Corn
Dried Beans
Dried Peas
Lima Beans
White Potato
Sweet Potato
Yams

25% Fruits - 5 - 12 oz. daily requirement.
Only 10 to 20% citrus. If canned, use only water packed or pour off syrup. Raw best, then frozen, then canned. Try mix-

233

ing with plain (homemade, if possible)
yogurt for fruit salad. Avoid after 6 PM.

5% Natural Sugar

Cantaloupe
Honey Dew
Rhubarb
Strawberries
Watermelon

15% Natural Sugar

Apples
Blueberries
Cherries
Grapes
Kumquats
Loganberries
Pears
Pineapple
Raspberries

10% Natural Sugar

Apricots
Blackberries
Cranberries
Currants
Grapefruit
Lemons
Limes
Oranges
Peaches
Plums

20% Natural Sugar

Bananas
Grape Juice
Fresh Prunes
Raisins
Dates
Figs

Food from this list should make up approximately
70% of your daily diet by weight. The following foods
can be used to make up the rest of your diet:

15% Starch - 3 - 8 oz. daily requirement. Determined
by activity.

Grains

Whole Grain Bread
Whole Grain Cereal
Brown Rice
Millet
Granola, Grapenuts
Bran

Potatoes

White   (All baked or
Yellow   Broiled)
Yams

Hollywood Bread
Occasional Tacos
Vegetarian Pizza

10% Protein - Fat - 2 - 4 oz. daily requirement.
Raw Seeds: Sunflower, pumpkin
Raw Sprouts: Alfalfa, Beans, Grains
Raw Nuts: Almonds, Cashews, etc.
Raw Eggs: (in drinks) or poached soft
Raw Milk, if possible: limit 1 glass/day
or yogurt, plain

Occasionally use (1-2x/week) in order
of preference:
Cheese: from natural food stores
(least additives) or brick such as
Colby, M. Jack
Fish: with scales, e.g., pike, haddock,
walleye, redsnapper, etc.
Chicken: no skin
Turkey: no skin
Lamb: no fat
Beef: no fat

Foods Prohibited

Spaghetti, macaroni, white rice
Pie, cake, pastry, sugar, candy
(Use raw honey sparingly for sweetening, sorghum,
pure maple syrup, or unsulphured blackstrap molasses.)
Carbonated cola and other soft drinks. (Use herb teas
and distilled water)
Alcohol in all forms.
Salt (try using herbs)
Coffee, tea (regular) Not more than 1 cup daily, unless
used as an enema.

Get in the habit of reading labels even in natural
food stores.

Energy Equivalents Chart

Number of minutes required at the activities listed to expend the caloric energy of food items shown below.

		Caloric Content	Reclining	Walking	Bicycle Riding	Swimming	Running
Beverages, Nonalcoholic	Carbonated, 8 oz. glass	106	82	20	13	9	5
	Ice cream soda, chocolate	255	196	49	31	23	13
	Malted milk shake, chocolate	502	386	97	61	45	26
	Milk, 8 oz. glass	166	128	32	20	15	9
	Milk, skim, 8 oz. glass	81	62	16	10	7	4
	Milk shake, chocolate	421	324	81	51	38	22
Desserts	Cake, 2-layer, 1/12	356	274	68	43	32	18
	Cookie, chocolate chip	51	39	10	6	5	3
	Doughnut	151	116	29	18	13	8
	Ice cream, 1/6 qt.	193	148	37	24	17	10
	Gelatin, with cream	117	90	23	14	10	6
	Pie, apple, 1/6	377	290	73	46	34	19
	Sherbet, 1/6 qt.	177	136	34	22	16	9
	Strawberry shortcake	400	308	77	49	36	21
Meats	Bacon, 2 strips	96	74	18	12	9	5
	Ham, 2 slices	167	128	32	20	15	9
	Pork chop, loin	314	242	60	38	28	16
	Steak, T-bone	235	181	45	29	21	12

Poultry & Eggs	Chicken, fried, 1/2 breast	232	178	45	28	21	12
	Chicken, "TV-Dinner"	542	217	104	66	48	28
	Turkey, 1 slice	130	100	25	16	12	7
	Egg, fried	110	85	21	13	10	6
	Egg, boiled	77	59	15	9	7	4
Sandwiches & Snacks	Club	590	454	113	72	53	30
	Hamburger	350	269	67	43	31	18
	Roast beef, with gravy	430	331	83	52	38	22
	Tunafish salad	278	214	53	34	25	14
	Pizza, with cheese, 1/8	180	138	35	22	16	9
	Potato chips, 1 serving	108	83	21	13	10	6
	Cheddar cheese, 1 oz.	111	85	21	14	10	6
Seafood	Clams, 6 medium	100	77	19	12	9	5
	Cod, steamed, 1 piece	80	62	15	10	7	4
	Crabmeat, 1/2 cup	68	52	13	8	6	4
	Haddock, 1 piece	71	55	14	9	6	4
	Halibut steak, 1/4 lb.	205	158	39	25	18	11
	Lobster, 1 medium	50	38	10	6	4	3
	Shrimp, french-fried, 1 serving	180	138	35	22	16	9

continued on next page

continued from preceding page

Number of minutes required at the activities listed to expend the caloric energy of food items shown below.

		Caloric Content	Reclining	Walking	Bicycle Riding	Swimming	Running
Miscellaneous	Bread & butter, 1 slice	78	60	15	10	7	4
	Cereal, dry 1/2 cup, with milk, sugar	200	154	38	24	18	10
	French dressing, 1 tbsp.	59	45	11	7	5	3
	Mayonnaise, 1 tbsp.	92	71	18	11	8	5
	Pancake, with syrup	124	95	24	15	11	6
	Spaghetti, 1 serving	396	305	76	48	35	20
	Cottage cheese, 1 tbsp.	27	21	5	3	2	1
Fruits & Fruit Juices	Apple, large	101	78	19	12	9	5
	Banana, small	88	68	17	11	8	4
	Orange, medium	68	52	13	8	6	4
	Peach, medium	46	35	9	6	4	2
	Apple juice, 8 oz. glass	118	91	23	14	10	6
	Orange juice, 8 oz. glass	120	92	23	15	11	6
	Tomato juice, 8 oz. glass	48	37	9	6	4	2
Vegetables	Beans, green, 1 cup	27	21	5	3	2	1
	Beets, canned, 1/2 cup	38	29	7	5	3	2
	Carrot, raw	42	32	8	5	4	2
	Lettuce, 3 large leaves	30	23	6	4	3	2
	Peas, green, 1/2 cup	56	43	11	7	5	3
	Potato, boiled, 1 medium	100	77	19	12	9	5
	Spinach, fresh, 1/2 cup	20	15	4	2	2	1

ADDED HELP

Fasting is a lot easier than it used to be. God has given us a tremendous breakthrough. We can go without food for 10 days and experience no hunger at all. In the process of looking for a good internal cleanser, I came across one that took away all hunger. I have since added it to our weight loss program and call it. . ."The Fasting Powder."

The fasting powder is made from herbs and seeds. You stir a rounded teaspoonful into a glass of water and drink it down. I think it tastes fine, but you might not. In that case, use a 16 oz. glass of water rather than an 8 oz. glass to dilute the taste. By the way, drink it down quickly. Don't give it a chance to gel. It's hard to drink once it gels.

The fasting powder has vitamins and minerals which are good to have when fasting. There are only 5 calories per teaspoon, so there's no danger of triggering any hunger. The powder was developed by a Christian doctor and I'm so delighted with it, I plan to take it for the rest of my life.

This same Christian doctor also introduced me to Bernard Jensen's BROTH. It is made of uncooked raw vegetables with a nice vitamin and mineral balance and has almost no calories. It won't trigger any hunger and it sure tastes great after you've gone without food for a few days. I've used it a number of times, especially before going to bed. It makes me feel as though I've had a bowl of soup. Go easy on the broth. Start with 1/2 teaspoon and increase it to your liking. Somewhere between 1/2 and 3/4 is just right for me.

Now that we can fast for 10 days with no hunger, we have the necessary dynamite for blasting Satan's food stronghold and that clears the way for installing the NEW IMAGE in our minds. This is the part that really gets the job done, but please see that we can't even get to this step without first subduing our flesh with a fast.

HINT: If you've never fasted before and feel hesitant, you may wish to ease into your first fast. Start on Monday and go for one day. Eat normally for the next 2 days, then start another fast and this time go for 2 days. Then eat normally for the next 2 days and go on a third fast, this time for 3 days. This will put you beyond the hunger stage. If you still haven't satisfied yourself that you can fast safely, then go on a 4 day fast. After 4 days of fasting, you'll know what fasting is all about. In this way, you can work yourself up to a 10 day fast.

To make your first fast easy, I have prepared a 4th cassette that takes you through the whole ten days. Actually, we go on the fast together. The cassette is called. . .FASTING MADE EASY and is included in the Christian weight loss package, which has a total of 7 items: the book, Help Lord, the Devil Wants Me Fat! 4 cassettes, the fasting powder and the broth. This gives you everything you need to get that weight off with no hunger. Write or call for free information on the package and a catalog of all of Dr. Lovett's works.

PERSONAL CHRISTIANITY
BOX 549, BALDWIN PARK, CA 91706
(818) 338-7333